COOKING FOR *Life*

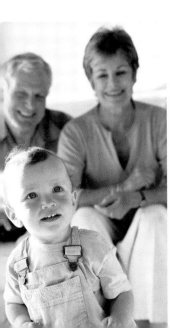

RECIPES

FOR

HEALTHY

LIVING

VOLUME 2

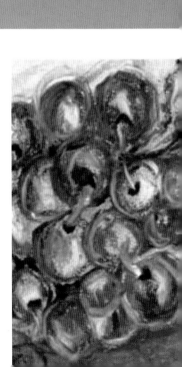

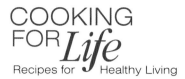

COOKING FOR *Life*

Recipes for Healthy Living

Published by Avera McKennan Foundation

Copyright © 2006 by
Avera McKennan Foundation
800 East 21st Street
Sioux Falls, South Dakota 57105

This cookbook is a collection of favorite recipes,
which are not necessarily original recipes.

Library of Congress Catalog Number: 2005905151
ISBN: 0-9760598-1-9

Edited and Manufactured by
Favorite Recipes® Press
An imprint of

FRP

P.O. Box 305142
Nashville, Tennessee 37230
800-358-0560

Art Director: Steve Newman
Project Editor: Debbie Van Mol, RD

First Printing: 2006   7,500 copies

Printed in China

Contributors

Project Managers: Tina Ames
                                Ann Carroll

Recipe Development: Nikki Ver Steeg, RD, LN

Recipe Editors: Nikki Ver Steeg, RD, LN
Joanne Shearer, RD, MS, CDE, LN
Food Service Team of the Avera Heart
    Hospital of South Dakota

Contributing Editors: Natalie Eidsness
Mary Michaels

Project Advisor: Jennifer Cisar

Book Design: Henkin Schultz Communication Arts

Illustrations and
   Photography: ©Henkin Schultz Communication Arts

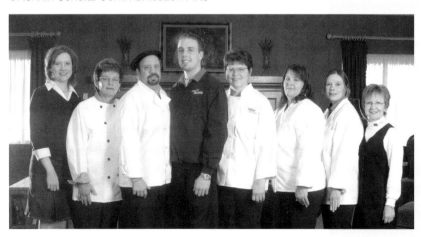

Left-right above: Nikki Ver Steeg, RD, LN; Donna Puthoff, Chef;
Al Flanigan, Chef; Jason Ruckelshausen, Food Service Assistant;
Mary Griffin, Chef; Brenda Kientopf, Chef; Kay Billam, Chef;
Joanne Shearer, RD, LN.

The workings of the human heart are the profoundest mystery of the universe. We see in them the reflection of the divine image.

—Charles W. Chestnut 1858–1899

This window in the Avera Heart Hospital Chapel was a gift from the Benedictine and Presentation Sisters in honor of the hospital's first anniversary. The gift celebrates the extension of the Sisters' health ministry at the Avera Heart Hospital. The window, created by artist Ken Bird of Sioux Falls, represents the diverse South Dakota landscape—from farmland and rolling plains in the east to the pine-covered Black Hills in the west.

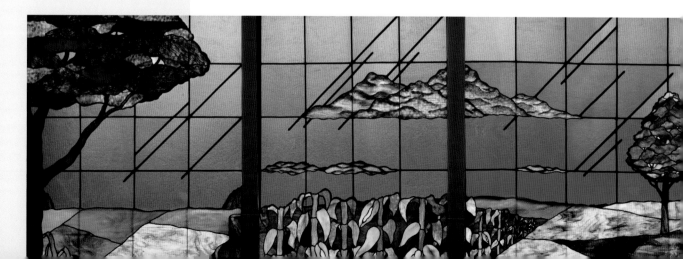

Contents

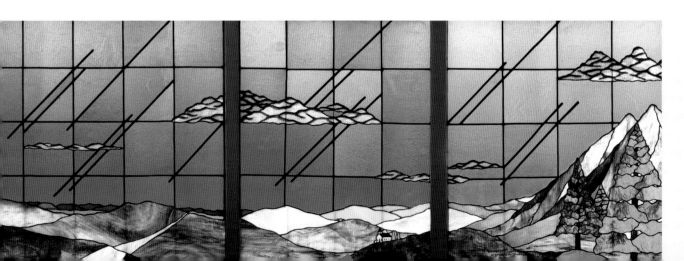

Foreword

Mark Twain once wrote, "The only way to keep your health is to eat what you don't want, drink what you don't like, and do what you'd rather not." As a registered dietitian, licensed nutritionist, and someone who enjoys eating, I can tell you that Mr. Twain never tried recipes like the ones found in the second volume of COOKING FOR LIFE!

Committing to a heart-healthy diet does not mean sacrificing the enjoyment that comes from sitting down to a delicious meal. This volume of COOKING FOR LIFE focuses on recipes designed to help you make food choices that are as good tasting as they are good for you. This collection of recipes is an opportunity to nourish your family while teaching the importance of a healthy diet.

What I really like about this cookbook is that it provides recipes that soon become family favorites—whether you are cooking for someone with heart disease, or just want to keep yourself and loved ones healthy. Live long, live better—start COOKING FOR LIFE.

To Your Health,

Nikki Ver Steeg, RD, LN
Clinical Nutrition Specialist
Avera Heart Hospital of South Dakota

Preface

Mealtime. Just the thought of sitting down to a great meal with your family seems to warm your heart. With the help of COOKING FOR LIFE, VOLUME 2, mealtime may also help save your heart. For millions of people who have experienced a heart attack or have battled conditions like high blood pressure or high cholesterol, a heart-healthy diet is essential. But being heart-smart is important for everyone, no matter what age or level of health.

Food and nutrition specialists from Avera Heart Hospital of South Dakota and Avera McKennan agree that starting a heart-healthy diet early in life can prevent heart disease and other health complications. This is why a team of dietitians, chefs, and other health specialists at Avera Heart Hospital of South Dakota have produced COOKING FOR LIFE, VOLUME 2. This cookbook focuses on making it easy for you to nourish those you love with meals that you've prepared from the heart—for the heart.

Mealtime...now the heart-warming time you spend with your family at the table can also be heart-saving. COOKING FOR LIFE, VOLUME 2, focuses on making it easy for you to nourish those you love with meals that you've prepared from the heart—for the heart.

The Avera Heart Hospital of South Dakota

♡ Skilled, Compassionate Care That Is State-of-the-Heart

At the Avera Heart Hospital of South Dakota, we focus our resources on heart and vascular disease. How to fight it. How to beat it.

For patients we offer hope, compassion, and a comprehensive approach to keeping the heart healthy and treating it when it's not. For physicians, we are a powerful resource, specially designed and equipped to support the cardiovascular caregiver in the pursuit of a better way to provide heart care.

Our physicians are empowered to make medical decisions that implement their best judgment on behalf of the patient. We practice "Patient Focused Care," a concept that includes assigning a team of six to eight highly trained caregivers to follow patients throughout their stay. This intimate approach promotes understanding, bonding, and continuity of care. All of our patient rooms are private and fully equipped to meet the special needs of heart patients.

♡ Recognized Chest Pain Center

The Avera Heart Hospital of South Dakota is accredited as a Chest Pain Center by the Society of Chest Pain Centers. The Society provides guidelines for treatment for patients with chest pain, which positively impacts the management of heart attack patients by improving patient outcomes and saving lives.

Achieving this accreditation demonstrates our dedication to the pursuit of excellence in the treatment of Acute Coronary Syndrome (ACS). It is important to understand that chest pain is often a serious sign of underlying ACS and should be treated as such. Any person who experiences chest pain should call an ambulance and get to the nearest Emergency Department for assessment and treatment.

This accreditation provides assurance that the facility has the systems, equipment, and people to treat patients with chest pain. An internal medicine physician and specially trained nursing staff are in our Emergency Department twenty-four hours a day, seven days a week. The cardiologists of North Central Heart are also available, either in the hospital or nearby, twenty-four hours a day.

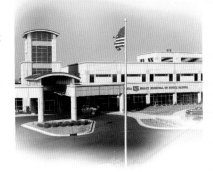

♡ Personalized Nutrition with Outpatient Nutrition Counseling

The recipes in this book will get you on your way to a heart-healthy diet. If you need additional assistance in developing a nutrition plan that works for you and your lifestyle, our Registered Dietitians can help.

The outpatient nutrition counseling program includes a meeting with an Avera Heart Hospital Registered Dietitian, a review of your current food intake, and a customized nutrition plan based on results of current blood work (including lipid panel and blood sugar), genetics, and existing medical conditions. We also evaluate your dietary supplements for adequacy and any interactions with foods or other medications you take. Taking this step can help with such conditions as:

- High blood pressure
- Diabetes
- Polycystic ovarian syndrome
- Coronary artery disease
- Reflux and heartburn
- Osteoporosis
- Kidney disease
- High cholesterol
- Overweight
- Metabolic syndrome
- Irritable bowel
- Fibromyalgia
- Chronic constipation
- Cancer
- Autoimmune Disease

The Avera Heart Hospital of South Dakota is a cooperative venture between Avera McKennan Hospital and University Health Center, North Central Heart Institute, and MedCath, Inc. For more information about nutrition counseling and other services, call 605-977-7000 or visit www.southdakotaheart.com.

Avera Heart Hospital Quick Facts

- Laboratory on site
- Pharmacy on site
- Full radiology department
- Respiratory therapy
- Chapel

Our comprehensive medical staff of more than 200 physicians represents specialties in the areas of pulmonology, nephrology, pathology, radiology, anesthesiology, family physicians, internists, vascular surgeons, cardiology, emergency, urology, and general surgeons.

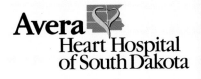

Avera Heart Hospital of South Dakota

The Heart-Healthy Diet

Commonly Asked Questions

What about the margarines that are advertised as helping lower cholesterol? Should I spend the extra money for those? The main difference with these margarines is the presence of stanols and sterols, natural plant compounds found in a variety of foods. If you have elevated LDL cholesterol, the extra cost of getting stanols and sterols is well worth the investment. A daily intake of two grams per day of stanols or sterols combined with a heart-healthy diet can reduce LDL cholesterol by 20 percent.

What's the difference between light olive oil and extra-virgin olive oil? Extra-virgin olive oil has more nutritional value than the light olive oil. Because extra-virgin olive oil is made from the first pressing of the olives, more heart-healthy plant compounds are retained in the oil.

Which cheese is best? Regular cheeses are high in saturated fats and need to be limited on a heart-healthy diet. There are many tasty low-fat cheeses now available in supermarkets. Mozzarella cheese and farmer cheese are naturally low in fat. Soy cheeses have no saturated fats or cholesterol. Using just a small amount of strong-flavored cheeses, like extra-sharp Cheddar cheese, fresh Parmesan cheese, or blue cheese, boosts flavor with a minimal amount of saturated fats.

Is regular ground beef allowable if rinsed after browning? Rinsing regular ground beef with hot water after cooking does remove some of the saturated fat. However, high-fat ground beef may actually be more expensive per pound after you consider cooking losses. Your best bet, both nutritionally and economically, is to buy the extra-lean ground beef. Even better, replace some of the ground beef with soy crumbles.

How much salt is recommended? The American Heart Association and the US Dietary Guidelines recommend a limit of 2,300 milligrams of sodium per day. This equates to the amount of sodium found in one teaspoon of salt. The majority of salt in the Standard American Diet is "hidden" salt.

In fact, a whopping 75 percent of the sodium in the American diet comes from processed, packaged, and canned foods. Only 15 percent comes from salt added at the table. Read food labels, and limit those packaged foods that have more than 250 milligrams of sodium per serving.

How much caffeine is allowable if you have heart disease? Most heart patients can drink regular coffee in moderation, or two to three cups per day. However, if you have an irregular heartbeat, you will want to avoid caffeine altogether. This includes regular coffee, soft drinks with caffeine, and regular tea.

Can I take flax oil tablets and get the same benefit as from ground flax? Ground flax gives you a bigger nutritional punch than just consuming flax oil. Flax oil is missing the fiber, vitamins, minerals, and cancer-protective nutrients found in ground flaxseed. And the cholesterol-lowering benefits of flaxseed are primarily from the fiber, not the oil. In addition, the magnesium and potassium in the ground flax helps with lowering blood pressure.

I get fish burps from my fish oil capsules. Any suggestions to combat this? Be sure to buy a high-quality fish oil that is certified for purity, potency, and freshness. Take with meals and in divided doses. If you still have stomach upset, store fish oil capsules in the freezer and take directly from the freezer.

Are fish oils contaminated with mercury? How do I know the fish oil supplement is safe? The good news is that most fish oil supplements on the market are free of mercury contamination, according to an independent laboratory that tests supplements for purity and quality. Out of twenty popular brands of fish oil supplements, Consumer Labs found NO detectable amounts of mercury. Most of the mercury is concentrated in the fish meat, not the oil, and the distillation process removes the contaminants. The Natural Pharmacist (www.tnp.com) provides additional information about fish oil supplements.

I am confused with all of the various vitamins on the market. How do I know if my vitamin is a good one? Look for a full spectrum multivitamin and mineral supplement that contains 100 percent of the Daily Value for nutrients. Because some nutrients are bulky, such as calcium and magnesium, it's not possible to pack every nutrient into a single pill. You may need to take several pills to get all of your essential nutrients at the 100 percent Daily Value. Look for the USP symbol on the label to ensure the vitamin disintegrates within thirty to forty-five minutes. Check with your dietitian, physician, or pharmacist regarding nutritional supplement and drug interactions.

Nutrition for Life

Live longer, live better.

The Avera Heart Hospital of South Dakota's diet approach for the prevention and treatment of cardiovascular disease is a modified Mediterranean approach, called the Prairie Mediterranean Diet. The Prairie Mediterranean Diet is based on the best components of the Mediterranean diet, combined with wholesome foods from the prairie. The Prairie Mediterranean Diet is more than a diet to prevent cardiovascular disease. This nutrition plan works for a range of conditions, including:

- Obesity
- Autoimmune and inflammatory diseases, diabetes, insulin resistance, and metabolic syndrome
- Depression and mental disorders
- Allergies and skin conditions, such as eczema and psoriasis
- COPD
- Crohn's disease and ulcerative colitis

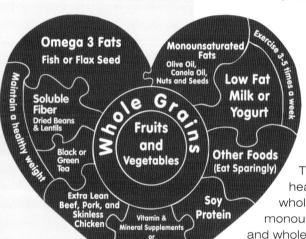

Omega 3 Fats
Fish or Flax Seed

Monounsaturated Fats
Olive Oil, Canola Oil, Nuts and Seeds

Exercise 3-5 times a week

Low Fat Milk or Yogurt

Maintain a healthy weight

Soluble Fiber
Dried Beans & Lentils

Whole Grains

Fruits and Vegetables

Black or Green Tea

Other Foods
(Eat Sparingly)

Extra Lean Beef, Pork, and Skinless Chicken

Soy Protein

Vitamin & Mineral Supplements or Foods Fortified with Folic Acid, B6 and B12

There is no single magical food you can eat to prevent heart disease. The Prairie Mediterranean Diet combines whole grains, legumes, fruits and vegetables, monounsaturated fats, soy foods, Omega-3 fatty acids, fiber, and whole grains to significantly decrease your risk of heart disease and keep you healthy.

Know your cholesterol numbers.

It is important that you know your cholesterol numbers. Different foods will affect different lipid fractions (lipid is just another name for fat). For example, saturated fats and trans fats raise LDL cholesterol ("lousy" cholesterol), while processed refined carbohydrates raise triglycerides. Below is a chart that defines the various lipid fractions and the target goal for each.

Lipid fraction	Goal	Definition	Foods that increase	Foods that decrease
LDL cholesterol	Less than 130 Less than 100 if you have heart disease	"Lousy" cholesterol	Saturated fats, trans fats (stick margarine, shortening, fried foods); to a lesser amount– dietary cholesterol	Soluble fiber, monounsaturated fats, ground flax, soy protein
HDL cholesterol	Greater than 55	"Healthy" cholesterol	Omega-3 fats, monounsaturated fats	Refined carbohydrates; trans fats, vegetable oils
Triglycerides	Less than 150	Blood fats	White refined carbs, trans fats, sugars, regular pop, and fruit juices	Fish and fish oils, ground flax, soluble fiber

Follow the 90/10 rule when planning your food choices. Eat 90 percent of the time within the heart puzzle and less than 10 percent from "splurge" foods. If you want to have the highest heart protection, you should eat "splurge" foods only two to four times a week.

Fruits and Vegetables

There are many heart-healthy benefits of fruits and vegetables including:
- Lowers risk of stroke
- Reduces blood pressure
- Lowers cholesterol

It is important to choose a wide variety of colors and textures when choosing fruits and vegetables. Fruit juice is a processed form of the fruit; therefore, limit your intake and choose only 100 percent juice.

Phytochemicals (fight-o chemicals) fight to protect your heart

A phytochemical is a cousin of vitamins found in plant foods. Phytochemicals work with other nutrients to protect against heart disease. *Phyto* is a Greek word that means plant. Brightly colored fruits and vegetables, yellow, orange, red, green, blue, and purple, generally contain the most phytochemicals and the most heart-protective nutrients.

Folate and homocysteine

Fruits, vegetables, and dried beans are good sources of folate, a B vitamin that helps to lower homocysteine. Homocysteine is a bad amino acid formed from the breakdown of protein. Homocysteine, like cholesterol, causes plaque buildup. Getting plenty of folate from fruits and vegetables helps convert homocysteine to other amino acids that are not harmful. The best sources of folate are green leafy vegetables, asparagus, broccoli, dried beans, and peas. Other good sources of folate include oranges, sweet potatoes, cantaloupe, cauliflower, and red bell peppers.

Antioxidants protect LDLs

Antioxidants (vitamin E, vitamin C, selenium, beta carotene) in fruits and vegetables protect LDL, "lousy" cholesterol, from oxidation. Once LDL is oxidized, it is more likely to build up in your arteries as plaque.

Whole Grains vs. Processed Carbohydrates

Heart-healthy benefits of whole grains
- Lowers risk of heart attack
- Lowers cholesterol (soluble fibers)
- Reduces blood pressure
- May help prevent type 2 diabetes

Whole grains, such as quinoa, amaranth, kamut, millet, triticale, barley, and oats, include all three parts of the kernel: the bran, germ, and endosperm. Most of the heart-protective nutrients are found in the bran and germ layers. Unfortunately, the disease-fighting layers of the whole wheat kernels are removed during processing. You can spot whole grains in food products by looking for these key words on labels: whole wheat, cracked wheat, whole oats, and whole grain. In more than fifty studies, a high whole grain intake proved to lower the risk of heart disease and certain cancers. It takes only three servings of whole grains per day for a whopping 30 percent lower risk of heart disease.

Processed carbohydrates include white flour, white sugar, white rice, instant potatoes, cream of wheat, and refined cold cereals. Processed carbohydrates turn into blood sugar very rapidly, causing large releases of insulin. Excess blood insulin can increase clotting and risk of heart attack. Processed carbohydrates are high glycemic index carbohydrates and contribute to high triglyceride levels in the blood.

When choosing cold cereals, follow the 5/5 rule per serving:

- 5 grams or MORE fiber
- 5 grams or LESS sugar

Substituting Ground Flax in Baked Goods
3 tablespoons ground flax = 3 tablespoons flour + 1 tablespoon oil + 1 tablespoon liquid
1 tablespoon ground flax softened in 1/4 cup water = 1 egg

To preserve the highest amount of nutrients, store flaxseeds in the refrigerator after grinding and use within a few weeks. The heart health benefits you receive from ground flax seeds are mainly from the fiber; therefore, choose ground flax instead of flax oil pills.

Nutrition

Healthy Fats
Omega-3 fatty acids
Heart-healthy benefits of Omega-3 fatty acids
- Lowers risk of sudden death from heart attack
- Reduces risk of blood clots
- Smoothes out irregular heartbeats
- Reduces inflammation in blood vessels and helps conditions associated with inflammation: rheumatoid arthritis, asthma, Crohn's disease
- Lowers triglycerides (blood fats)
- Lowers blood pressure
- Increases HDL "healthy" cholesterol
- Improves depression
- Improves diabetic control by making cells more sensitive to insulin
- Improves allergies
- Helps autoimmune diseases: multiple sclerosis, lupus, psoriasis, type 1 diabetes
- Good for dry skin, dermatitis, and thinning hair

Are you surprised at all the wonderful health *benefits* of eating fats? It's true. Omega-3 fatty acids are a very important part of your heart-healthy diet.

There are several ways to incorporate Omega-3 fatty acids into your diet.

Animal sources of Omega-3 fatty acids
- **Best**—fatty fish such as salmon, herring, sardines, or tuna. Eat two servings of fatty fish a week. If you do not eat fish, you may take one fish oil capsule per day. If you take blood thinning medications, please check with your doctor before taking fish oil capsules.
- **Good**—Omega-3-enhanced eggs contribute significant amounts of Omega-3 fatty acids to your diet.
- **Fair**—Range-fed beef, wild game, purslane, and leafy greens.

Plant sources of Omega-3 fatty acids
- **Best**—Ground flaxseed. You can get your recommended amount of plant-based Omega fats by eating one tablespoon of ground flaxseeds per day.
- **Good**—Canola oil.
- **Fair**—Walnuts, soy protein (tofu, soy nuts).

Choosing a Better Oil
- Extra-virgin olive oil and canola oil are high in heart-healthy monounsaturated fats. Nuts, seeds, and nut butters are also excellent sources of monounsaturated fats.
- Extra-virgin refers to the first pressing of the olives. This olive oil has a high amount of heart-protective nutrients.
- Canola oil has a lighter, more bland flavor than olive oil and is more desirable for baking. Extra-virgin olive oil has a stronger taste and adds flavor to stir-fries and salads.

Substitute monounsaturated fats for some of the carbohydrates in your diet. Instead of cookies, graham crackers, popcorn, or pretzels for snacks, eat a handful of soy nuts, walnuts, almonds, or sunflower seed kernels. Eliminate bread or starch at the evening meal and have a salad with olive oil and vinegar dressing.

Nutrition

Dairy and Lean Protein

Heart-healthy benefits of low-fat milk and yogurt:

- Reduces blood pressure
- Helps with weight control
- Lowers cholesterol (yogurt)

Lean protein

Extra-lean beef and pork are allowable on a heart-healthy diet in controlled portions. Beef, pork, and poultry are excellent sources of B vitamins, protein, iron, zinc, and selenium. Look for "loin" and "round" for the leanest cuts of beef and pork.

Saturated fats—eat sparingly

Fatty meats and poultry skin are high in saturated fats that increase your LDL (lousy) cholesterol. Fatty meats and full-fat dairy products are the highest sources of saturated fats. You can limit saturated fats by eating very lean meat, wild game, poultry without the skin, and low-fat dairy products.

Tea

Heart-healthy benefits of tea

- Protects LDL from oxidation
- Lowers cholesterol
- Lowers risk of fatal heart attack
- Increases HDL "healthy" cholesterol

Other health benefits

- Helps prevent cancer
- Improves immunity
- Reduces stress

Rich in nutrients like phytochemicals, antioxidants, and flavonoids, tea can actually reduce the risk of fatal heart attack. Fresh brewed tea provides more heart-healthy phytochemicals than iced tea mixes or bottled drinks. In addition, green tea is closest to its natural form and provides the most flavonoids per serving.

Soluble Fiber

Heart-healthy benefits of soluble fiber
- Helps lower blood pressure
- Lowers total and LDL cholesterol (soluble fiber)
- Potential to lower homocysteine

Dried beans–a perfect heart-healthy food

Dried beans pack a huge nutritional punch.
- Highest food sources of fiber, both insoluble and soluble.
- They are loaded with vitamins, minerals, and phytochemicals.
- A low-cost source of protein.

Soluble fiber in dried beans forms a gel in your intestines that blocks the absorption of bile salts. This in turn prevents absorption of cholesterol. Besides heart benefits, soluble fiber helps control blood sugars by slowing down the absorption of carbohydrates.

Canned beans have the same nutritional value as beans prepared from the dried state. Rinse canned beans before using them to lower the sodium level.

Nutrition

Soy

Heart-healthy benefits of soy foods
- Reduction in total cholesterol
- Reduction in LDL cholesterol
- Lowers triglycerides
- Lowers blood pressure
- Protects LDL from oxidation

Other health benefits
- Associated with lower cancer risk
- May help with blood sugar control in diabetics
- Easier on the kidneys than animal protein
- May reduce menopausal symptoms

Besides being a good source of protein, soybeans are a great source of fiber, vitamin E, and Omega-3 fatty acids. Soybeans have a low glycemic index, meaning the carbohydrates in soybeans are slowly absorbed as sugar.

Danger Zone

There is NO safe intake of the following artery-clogging fats.

Trans or hydrogenated fats

Trans fats are formed during the processing of vegetable oils into solid fat. Food manufacturers add hydrogen to oil to make it solid. Trans fats are often found in solid stick margarine, shortening, fried foods, fast foods, microwave popcorn, store-bought cookies and crackers, cakes, and pastries. Trans fats increase LDL cholesterol and lower HDL levels. Trans fats worsen insulin resistance, which in turn contributes to higher triglycerides.

The Food and Drug Administration has mandated that food manufacturers add trans fat information to the food fact label by the year 2006. Choose those foods that have no more than one gram of trans fats per serving. Check out the ingredient label. If you see the term "partially hydrogenated oil," this is a telltale sign for trans fats.

To convert from the Standard American Diet (SAD) to the Prairie Mediterranean Diet:

- Increase fruits and vegetables to 8 servings per day.

- Replace saturated and hydrogenated fats with monounsaturated fats.

- Add Omega-3 fats to your diet from fish, flax, canola oil, and walnuts.

- Choose quality carbohydrates from whole grains, fruits, vegetables, beans, and lentils.

- Limit processed packaged foods, especially those with hydrogenated fats.

- Increase soluble fiber sources from barley, oats, beans, lentils, sweet potatoes, and fruits.

- Add one to two servings of soy foods daily to your diet.

- Use portion control for weight control.

- Incorporate exercise into your daily routine.

For every 2 percent increase in calories from trans fatty acids, there is over a 90 percent increase in heart disease. Just eating one doughnut for breakfast and a large order of French fries for lunch provides 5 percent of calories from trans fats on a 2,000 calorie diet.

Nutritional Profile
Guidelines

The editors have attempted to present these family recipes in a format that allows approximate nutritional values to be computed. Persons with dietary or health problems or whose diets require close monitoring should not rely solely on the nutritional information provided. They should consult their physician or a registered dietitian for specific information.

Abbreviations for Nutritional Profile

CAL—Calories
PROT—Protein
CARBO—Carbohydrates
T FAT—Total Fat
SAT. FAT—Saturated Fat
MONOUFA—
   Monounsaturated Fatty Acids
FIBER—Dietary Fiber

SOD—Sodium
OMEGA-3 FA—
   Omega-3 Fatty Acids
Mg—Magnesium
K—Potassium
G—grams
MG—milligrams

Nutritional information for these recipes is computed from information derived from many sources, including materials supplied by the United States Department of Agriculture, computer databanks, and journals in which the information is assumed to be in the public domain. However, many specialty items, new products, and processed foods may not be available from these sources or may vary from the average values used in these profiles. More information on new and/or specific products may be obtained by reading the nutrient labels. Unless otherwise specified, the nutritional profile of these recipes is based on all measurements being level.

- Artificial sweeteners vary in use and strength and should be used to taste, using the recipe ingredients as a guideline. Sweeteners using aspartame (NutraSweet® and Equal®) should not be used as a sweetener in recipes involving prolonged heating, which reduces the sweet taste. For further information on the use of these sweeteners, refer to the package.
- Alcoholic ingredients have been analyzed for the basic information. Cooking causes the evaporation of alcohol, which decreases alcoholic and caloric content.
- Buttermilk, sour cream, and yogurt are the types available commercially.
- Canned beans and vegetables have been analyzed with the canning liquid. Rinsing and draining canned products will lower the sodium content.
- Chicken, cooked for boning and chopping, has been roasted; this method yields the lowest caloric values.
- Eggs are large Omega-3-enhanced. To avoid raw eggs that may carry salmonella, as in eggnog or six-week muffin batter, use eggs pasteurized in their shells, which are sold at some specialty food stores, or use an equivalent amount of pasteurized egg substitute.
- Flour is unsifted all-purpose flour.
- Garnishes, serving suggestions, and other optional information are not included in the profile.
- Margarine and butter are regular, not whipped or presoftened.
- Oil is either canola or olive.
- Salt and other ingredients to taste as noted in the ingredients have not been included in the nutritional profile.
- If a choice of ingredients has been given, the profile reflects the first option. If a choice of amounts has been given, the profile reflects the greater amount.

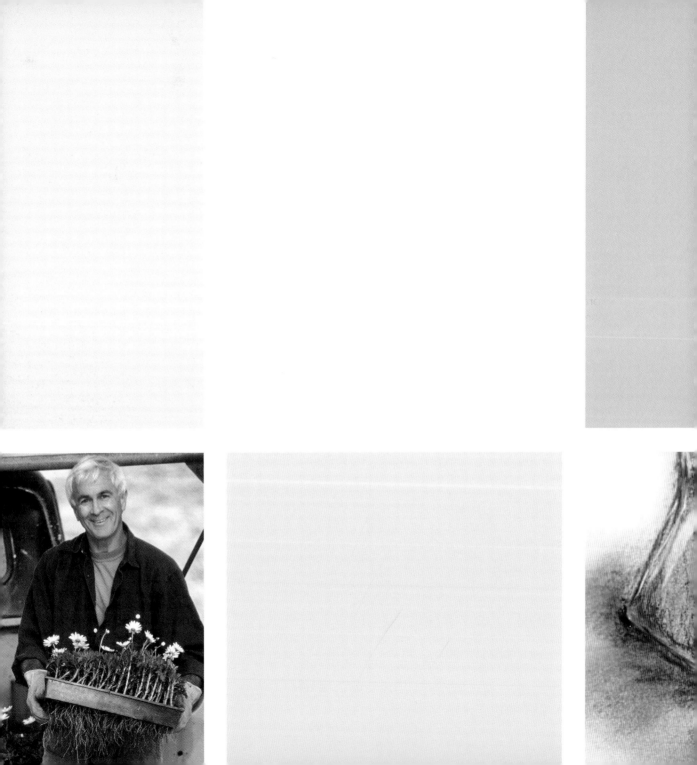

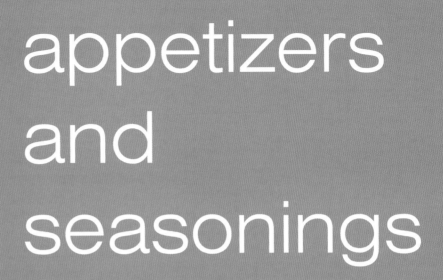

appetizers and seasonings

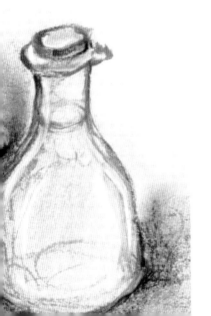

Appetizers and seasonings are like the opening lines of a good book—they set the tone for what is to follow. From salsa to shrimp, start your meal on a flavorful note. These recipes say "exotic" to friends and family, but they are simple to prepare.

appetizers

Mint Frost Coffee

2	cups skim milk	1	cup ice cubes
4	teaspoons instant coffee granules	2	tablespoons sugar
4	(2$^1/_3$-ounce) scoops lite vanilla ice cream	$^1/_8$	teaspoon peppermint extract

Combine the skim milk and coffee granules in a blender and process until the coffee dissolves. Add the ice cream, ice cubes, sugar and flavoring and process until smooth. Pour into glasses and serve immediately.

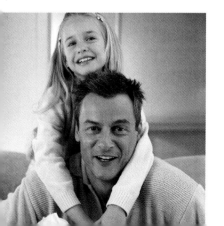

NUTRIENTS PER SERVING   Yield: 4 servings

CAL	PROT	CARBO	T FAT	SAT. FAT	MONOUFA	FIBER	SOD	OMEGA-3 FA	MG	K
188	7G	27G	5G	3G	<1G	0G	97MG	0G	16MG	223MG

Herb Cheese Dip

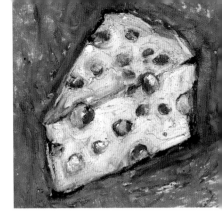

8	ounces part-skim ricotta cheese
3	ounces lite cream cheese, softened
1	tablespoon water
1/2	teaspoon lemon juice
2	teaspoons minced fresh parsley
2	teaspoons minced fresh dill weed, or 1/2 teaspoon dried dill weed
1/2	teaspoon crushed dried basil
1/2	teaspoon crushed dried tarragon
1	garlic clove, minced

Combine the ricotta cheese, cream cheese, water and lemon juice in a blender or food processor and process for 1 minute or until smooth. Add the parsley, dill weed, basil, tarragon and garlic and process for 30 seconds longer.

Spoon the dip into a bowl and chill, covered, in the refrigerator. Serve as a dip with raw vegetables or as a spread with Whole Wheat Crackers on page 34.

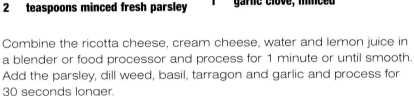

NUTRIENTS PER 2 TABLESPOONS   Yield: 12 (2-tablespoon) servings

CAL	PROT	CARBO	T FAT	SAT. FAT	MONOUFA	FIBER	SOD	OMEGA-3 FATS	MG	K
37	3G	1G	2G	1G	<1G	<1G	50MG	<1G	3MG	36MG

Curried Mayonnaise Dip

2/3 cup low-fat mayonnaise	**1/2** teaspoon turmeric
1/3 cup nonfat plain yogurt	**1/2** teaspoon chili powder
1 tablespoon curry powder	**1/2** teaspoon paprika
1 teaspoon ground ginger	**1/4** teaspoon salt

Combine the mayonnaise and yogurt in a bowl and mix well; do not whisk. Stir in the curry powder, ginger, turmeric, chili powder, paprika and salt. Chill, covered, in the refrigerator for 1 to 10 hours. Serve with raw vegetables, chips or Sweet Potato Strips on page 70.

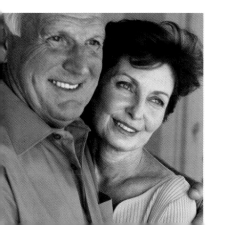

NUTRIENTS PER TABLESPOON								Yield: 16 (1-tablespoon) servings		
CAL	PROT	CARBO	T FAT	SAT. FAT	MONOUFA	FIBER	SOD	OMEGA-3 FA	MG	K
37	<1G	2G	3G	1G	<1G	<1G	120MG	0G	1MG	13MG

Black Bean **Salsa**

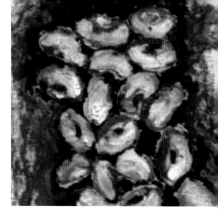

1	(8-ounce) can black beans, drained and rinsed	3	tablespoons low-sodium vegetable broth
8	ounces frozen corn, thawed and drained	3	tablespoons minced fresh cilantro
1	fresh tomato, chopped	3	tablespoons lime juice
3/4	cup chopped onion	2	garlic cloves, minced
1/2	cup chopped green bell pepper	1 1/2	teaspoons ground cumin

Combine the beans, corn, tomato, onion, bell pepper and broth in a bowl and mix well. Stir in the cilantro, lime juice, garlic and cumin. Serve with baked tortilla chips or as a side dish.

Besides lowering your risk of heart disease, the nutrients and fiber in beans and lentils protect against cancer, diseases of the colon, and diabetes.

NUTRIENTS PER 1/2 CUP   Yield: 6 (1/2-cup) servings

CAL	PROT	CARBO	T FAT	SAT. FAT	MONOUFA	FIBER	SOD	OMEGA-3 FATS	MG	K
84	4G	17G	1G	‹1G	‹1G	4G	123MG	‹1G	14MG	200MG

Feta-Stuffed Mushrooms

Choose extra-virgin olive oil or canola oil to help lower your LDL (bad cholesterol) and raise your HDL (good cholesterol).

2	pounds fresh small white mushrooms
3	tablespoons extra-virgin olive oil
1/3	cup chopped onion
2	teaspoons minced garlic
1/3	cup walnuts, chopped
1/2	teaspoon oregano
1/8	teaspoon ground pepper
4	ounces plain or seasoned feta cheese, crumbled

Remove the stems from the mushrooms and chop the stems. Toss the caps with 1 tablespoon of the olive oil in a bowl. Arrange the caps stem side down in a single layer in a shallow baking pan and bake at 400 degrees for 10 minutes or until tender. Maintain the oven temperature.

Heat the remaining 2 tablespoons olive oil in a small skillet over medium heat. Add the onion, garlic and reserved mushroom stems to the hot olive oil and cook for 5 minutes or until the stems are tender and the liquid evaporates, stirring constantly. Stir in the walnuts, oregano and pepper.

Spoon the walnut mixture into a bowl and blend in the cheese. Turn the mushroom caps over and mound the filling in the caps. Bake for 15 minutes or until heated through. Serve immediately.

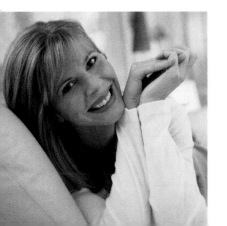

NUTRIENTS PER SERVING   Yield: 12 servings

CAL	PROT	CARBO	T FAT	SAT. FAT	MONOUFA	FIBER	SOD	OMEGA-3 FA	MG	K
96	5G	4G	7G	2G	3G	1G	106MG	‹1G	7MG	295MG

Marinated Tomatoes and Fresh Mozzarella

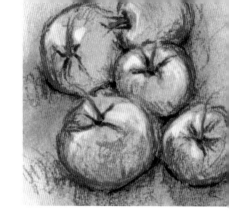

| 4 | tomatoes | **¹/₂** | **cup Balsamic Vinaigrette** |
| 1 | **pound fresh mozzarella cheese** | | **(page 61)** |

Cut each tomato into 4 equal slices. Cut the cheese into 16 thin slices. Top each tomato slice with 1 slice of the cheese and arrange the stacks on a large serving platter. Drizzle with the vinaigrette.

Chill, covered, in the refrigerator until serving time. Serve as an appetizer or as a sandwich garnish.

NUTRIENTS PER SERVING   Yield: 16 servings

CAL	PROT	CARBO	T FAT	SAT. FAT	MONOUFA	FIBER	SOD	OMEGA-3 FATS	MG	K
125	5G	3G	10G	5G	3G	‹1G	47MG	‹1G	5MG	93MG

Crunchy Baked Tomatoes

4	**large ripe tomatoes**
1	**tablespoon extra-virgin olive oil, or nonstick cooking spray**
3/4	**teaspoon salt**
1/2	**cup (2 ounces) shredded reduced-fat sharp Cheddar cheese**

1/2	**cup dry whole wheat bread crumbs**
1/2	**cup chopped dry-roasted peanuts**
2	**tablespoons unsalted butter or trans-fat-free margarine, melted**
3/4	**teaspoon basil**
1/8	**teaspoon cayenne pepper**

Cut the tomatoes into halves and lightly brush the outer surface with the olive oil. Arrange the tomato halves cut side up in a baking dish and sprinkle with the salt.

Combine the cheese, bread crumbs, peanuts, butter, basil and cayenne pepper in a bowl and mix well. Spoon about 1 heaping tablespoon of the cheese mixture on top of each tomato half and bake at 350 degrees for 15 minutes or until heated through.

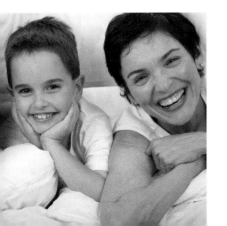

NUTRIENTS PER SERVING   Yield: 8 servings

CAL	PROT	CARBO	T FAT	SAT. FAT	MONOUFA	FIBER	SOD	OMEGA-3 FA	MG	K
134	5G	7G	11G	4G	4G	2G	240MG	‹1G	29MG	289MG

Spicy Shrimp

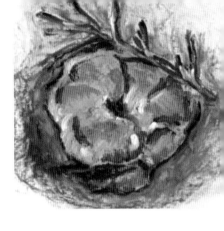

2	tablespoons extra-virgin olive oil
	Juice of 1 lemon
1	bay leaf
1	teaspoon crushed dried rosemary
1/2	teaspoon paprika
1/4	teaspoon cayenne pepper
1/8	teaspoon Tabasco sauce
1/8	teaspoon Worcestershire sauce
10	garlic cloves, minced
	Salt and freshly ground black pepper to taste
1 1/2	pounds (20 count) shrimp, peeled and deveined
	Chopped fresh parsley

Heat the olive oil in a heavy skillet over low heat. Stir in the lemon juice, bay leaf, rosemary, paprika, cayenne pepper, Tabasco sauce, Worcestershire sauce, garlic, salt and black pepper. Cook over low heat for 15 minutes, stirring occasionally. Increase the heat and stir in the shrimp.

Cook until the shrimp turn pink and begin to curl, swirling the pan constantly. Do not overcook. Spoon the shrimp mixture into a bowl and marinate, covered, in the refrigerator for 24 hours or longer. Discard the bay leaf and sprinkle with parsley before serving.

Trans fats are dangerous and result from partial hydrogenation. Limit your intake to lower your heart disease risk.

NUTRIENTS PER SERVING   Yield: 6 servings

CAL	PROT	CARBO	T FAT	SAT. FAT	MONOUFA	FIBER	SOD	OMEGA-3 FATS	MG	K
137	18G	2G	6G	1G	4G	<1G	196MG	<1G	31MG	187MG

Whole Wheat Crackers

Pair a protein and a carbohydrate together for snacks: trans-fat-free crackers with string cheese, natural peanut butter and an apple, a small handful of nuts, or one-half lean turkey sandwich on whole wheat bread.

1¹/2 cups whole wheat flour

1¹/2 cups all-purpose flour

¹/4 cup sugar

1 teaspoon salt

¹/2 teaspoon baking soda

¹/2 cup (1 stick) butter or trans-fat-free margarine, softened

³/4 cup buttermilk

¹/4 cup wheat germ

Sift the whole wheat flour, all-purpose flour, sugar, salt and baking soda together and add to a food processor. Add the butter and process until combined. Add the buttermilk and process until the mixture forms a ball. Let rest for 10 minutes. Divide the dough into 4 equal portions.

Coat 4 baking sheets with nonstick cooking spray and sprinkle each with 1 tablespoon of the wheat germ. Roll each dough portion to the desired thickness on 1 of the prepared baking sheets. Cut into the desired shapes with a pastry wheel.

Bake at 350 degrees for 20 to 25 minutes or until light brown. Cool on the baking sheets for 2 minutes and remove to a wire rack to cool completely. Store in an airtight container. Serve with Herb Cheese Dip on page 27.

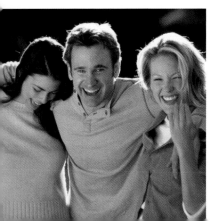

NUTRIENTS PER SERVING · Yield: 23 servings

CAL	PROT	CARBO	T FAT	SAT. FAT	MONOUFA	FIBER	SOD	OMEGA-3 FA	MG	K
107	3G	15G	4G	3G	1G	1G	166MG	<1G	17MG	67MG

Cajun Seasoning

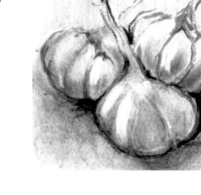

¹/₄ cup garlic powder	1¹/₂ teaspoons celery seeds
¹/₄ cup onion powder	1¹/₂ teaspoons chili powder
2 tablespoons paprika	1 teaspoon salt
1 tablespoon ground red pepper	1 teaspoon lemon pepper
1 tablespoon black pepper	¹/₂ teaspoon ground nutmeg

Combine the garlic powder, onion powder, paprika, red pepper, black pepper, celery seeds, chili powder, salt, lemon pepper and nutmeg in a jar with a tight-fitting lid and seal tightly. Shake to mix. Use as a rub for meat or fish, or to season your favorite dishes.

NUTRIENTS PER TEASPOON   Yield: 48 (1-teaspoon) servings

CAL	PROT	CARBO	T FAT	SAT. FAT	MONOUFA	FIBER	SOD	OMEGA-3 FATS	MG	K
7	<1G	1G	<1G	<1G	<1G	<1G	60MG	0G	2MG	27MG

Seasoning Salt

2   **tablespoons salt**   **1**   **tablespoon onion powder**

3   **tablespoons pepper**   **1**   **tablespoon garlic powder**

2   **tablespoons paprika**

Combine the salt, pepper, paprika, onion powder and garlic powder in a jar with a tight-fitting lid and seal tightly. Shake to mix. Use for seasoning beef, fish or chicken or sprinkle over potatoes before roasting.

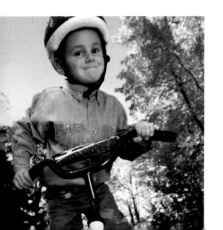

NUTRIENTS PER TEASPOON										Yield: 30 (1-teaspoon) servings
CAL	PROT	CARBO	T FAT	SAT. FAT	MONOUFA	FIBER	SOD	OMEGA-3 FA	MG	K
4	‹1G	1G	‹1G	‹1G	‹1G	‹1G	466MG	0G	2MG	23MG

South-of-the-Border
Seasoning

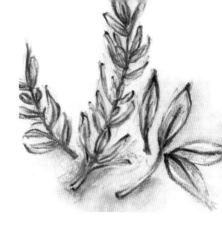

2	**tablespoons chili powder**	**1**	**tablespoon onion powder**
5	**teaspoons paprika**	**2¹/₂**	**teaspoons garlic powder**
4¹/₂	**teaspoons ground cumin**	**¹/₈**	**to ¹/₄ teaspoon cayenne pepper**

Combine the chili powder, paprika, cumin, onion powder, garlic powder and cayenne pepper in a jar with a tight-fitting lid and seal tightly. Shake to mix. This homemade version of taco seasoning is twice as spicy as the commercially-prepared version, so only add half as much to your favorite Mexican dishes.

Elevated homocysteine levels increase the risk for heart disease. Vitamins B6 and B12 and folic acid are homocysteine warriors that keep your levels under control.

NUTRIENTS PER TEASPOON   Yield: 16 (1-teaspoon) servings

CAL	PROT	CARBO	T FAT	SAT. FAT	MONOUFA	FIBER	SOD	OMEGA-3 FATS	MG	K
10	‹1G	2G	‹1G	‹1G	‹1G	1G	12MG	‹1G	4MG	43MG

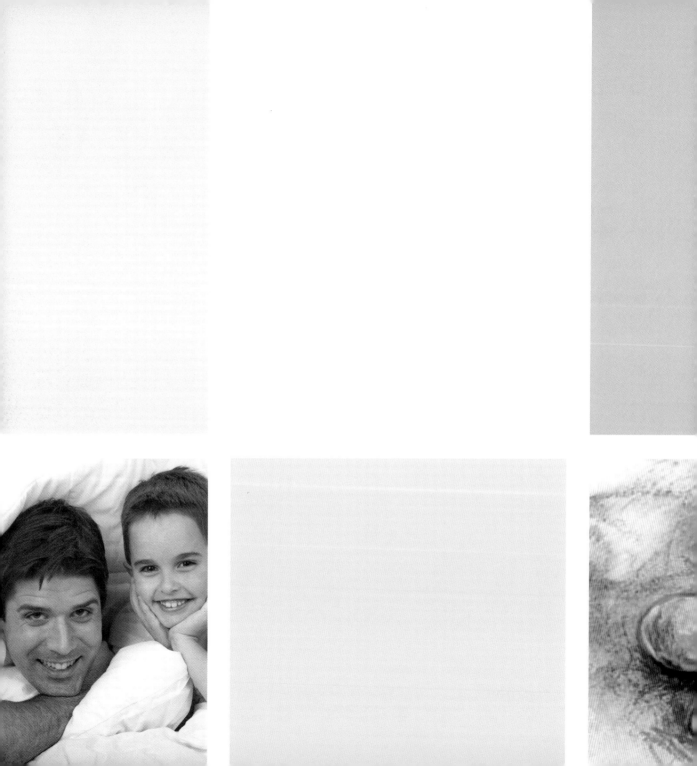

breakfast

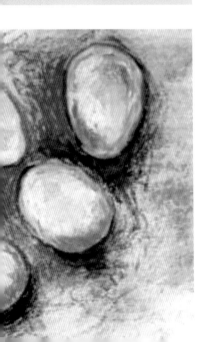

Not only is breakfast the most important meal of the day, but it can also be the most flavorful. Go beyond the cereal bowl with heart-healthy flax, Omega-3-enhanced eggs, and good-for-you fruits and nuts.

One cup of blueberries contains four grams of fiber. Blueberries are also a good source of vitamin C.

Super Soy Shake

3/4 **cup fresh or frozen blueberries**	1/6 **block (2.7 ounces) tofu**
3/4 **cup soy milk**	1 **tablespoon flaxseed, ground**
3/4 **cup orange juice**	1 **tablespoon wheat bran**
6 **to 8 baby carrots**	1 **tablespoon wheat germ**

Combine the blueberries, soy milk, orange juice, carrots, tofu, flaxseed, wheat bran and wheat germ in a blender and process until combined. Serve immediately.

NUTRIENTS PER SHAKE   Yield: 1 large shake

CAL	PROT	CARBO	T FAT	SAT. FAT	MONOUFA	FIBER	SOD	OMEGA-3 FATS	MG	K
416	22G	61G	13G	2G	2G	12MG	176MG	3G	164MG	1161MG

Cranberry Almond Granola

4 **cups old-fashioned oats**	1/4 **cup maple syrup**
1/4 **cup sliced almonds**	2 **teaspoons canola oil**
1/4 **cup ground flaxseed**	1/2 **teaspoon ground cinnamon**
1/4 **cup frozen orange juice concentrate, thawed**	1 1/3 **cups sweetened dried cranberries**

Mix the oats, almonds and flaxseed in a bowl. Whisk the orange juice concentrate, syrup, canola oil and cinnamon in a bowl and drizzle over the oat mixture, tossing until coated.

Spread the oat mixture evenly on 2 large baking sheets and bake at 325 degrees for 20 to 25 minutes or until light brown, stirring frequently. Stir in the cranberries and let stand until cool. Store in an airtight container.

NUTRIENTS PER 3/4 CUP   Yield: 8 (3/4-cup) servings

CAL	PROT	CARBO	T FAT	SAT. FAT	MONOUFA	FIBER	SOD	OMEGA-3 FA	MG	K
343	9G	61G	8G	1G	3G	7G	6MG	1G	96MG	329MG

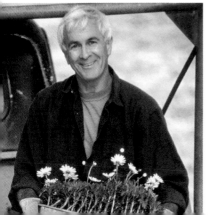

Cinnamon **Breakfast Bars**

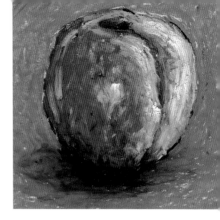

1/2 **cup chopped walnuts**	1 **cup oat bran cereal**
1 **tablespoon ground flaxseed**	1/4 **cup packed brown sugar**
1 **cup Bran Buds**	1 **teaspoon ground cinnamon**
1 1/4 **cups buttermilk**	1/2 **teaspoon salt**
1/4 **cup canola oil or applesauce**	1/2 **cup chopped dried apricots**
1 **Omega-3-enhanced egg**	2 **teaspoons granulated sugar**
1 **cup old-fashioned oats**	1 **teaspoon grated orange zest**

Toss the walnuts and flaxseed in a bowl and spread on a baking sheet lightly coated with nonstick cooking spray. Toast at 350 degrees for 5 to 7 minutes or until light brown, stirring occasionally. Remove to a platter to cool. Maintain the oven temperature.

Soften the Bran Buds in the buttermilk in a bowl for 10 minutes. Add the canola oil and egg and whisk until combined. Combine the oats, oat bran cereal, brown sugar, cinnamon, salt and walnut mixture in a bowl and mix well. Add the egg mixture to the oat mixture and mix well. Stir in the apricots, granulated sugar and orange zest.

Pour the cereal mixture into an 8x8-inch baking pan sprayed with nonstick cooking spray and bake for 20 to 30 minutes or until the edges pull from the sides of the pan. Let stand until cool and cut into bars. Store in an airtight container.

NUTRIENTS PER BAR   Yield: 1 dozen bars

CAL	PROT	CARBO	T FAT	SAT. FAT	MONOUFA	FIBER	SOD	OMEGA-3 FATS	MG	K
192	5G	25G	10G	1G	4G	5G	197MG	1G	50MG	286MG

Pecan **Power Bars**

3/4	cup honey	1/2	cup chopped pecans
1/4	cup canola oil	1	cup whole wheat flour
1	Omega-3-enhanced egg	1	cup old-fashioned oats
1	teaspoon vanilla extract	1/2	teaspoon baking soda
1	cup grated carrots	1/2	teaspoon salt
1	cup chopped pitted prunes	1/8	teaspoon ground allspice

Combine the honey, canola oil, egg and vanilla in a mixing bowl and beat until blended. Stir in the carrots, prunes and pecans. Combine the whole wheat flour, oats, baking soda, salt and allspice in a bowl and mix well. Stir the flour mixture into the honey mixture until incorporated.

Spread evenly in a 9x9-inch baking pan sprayed with nonstick cooking spray and bake at 350 degrees for 20 minutes. Let stand until cool and cut into 2x2-inch bars. Store in an airtight container.

For balance, be sure to include a protein with your breakfast.

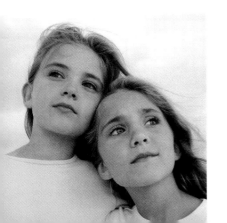

NUTRIENTS PER BAR
Yield: 1 dozen (2×2-inch) bars

CAL	PROT	CARBO	T FAT	SAT. FAT	MONOUFA	FIBER	SOD	OMEGA-3 FA	MG	K
237	4G	37G	9G	1G	5G	3G	163MG	1G	37MG	210MG

Apricot Cranberry Oatmeal

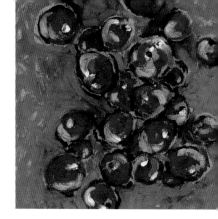

3³/₄ cups water

¹/₄ teaspoon salt

2 cups old-fashioned oats

¹/₂ cup sweetened dried cranberries

¹/₂ cup dried apricots, chopped

1 teaspoon ground cinnamon

1 cup skim milk

¹/₄ cup packed brown sugar

Bring the water and salt to a boil in a saucepan and stir in the oats, cranberries, apricots and cinnamon. Return to a boil and reduce the heat.

Simmer, covered, for 5 minutes or until thickened, stirring occasionally. Remove from the heat and let stand, covered, for 5 minutes. Stir in the skim milk and brown sugar just before serving.

NUTRIENTS PER SERVING — Yield: 4 servings

CAL	PROT	CARBO	T FAT	SAT. FAT	MONOUFA	FIBER	SOD	OMEGA-3 FATS	MG	K
352	10G	72G	4G	1G	1G	7G	180MG	‹1G	87MG	580MG

Turkey Sausage Patties

3	**pounds ground skinless extra-lean turkey breast**	**1¹/₂**	**teaspoons black pepper**
¹/₂	**cup unsweetened applesauce**	**1**	**teaspoon salt**
³/₄	**tablespoon sage**	**¹/₂**	**teaspoon red pepper flakes**
³/₄	**tablespoon thyme**	**¹/₂**	**teaspoon cayenne pepper**

Combine the ground turkey, applesauce, sage, thyme, black pepper, salt, red pepper flakes and cayenne pepper in a bowl and mix well. Shape the ground turkey mixture into twenty-four 2-ounce patties.

Cook the patties in a nonstick skillet over medium heat until cooked through and light brown on both sides. Serve immediately. You may freeze uncooked patties for future use. Cook from the frozen state.

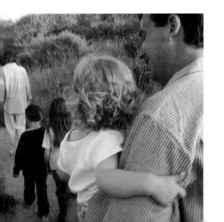

NUTRIENTS PER PATTY — Yield: 2 dozen patties

CAL	PROT	CARBO	T FAT	SAT. FAT	MONOUFA	FIBER	SOD	OMEGA-3 FA	MG	K
63	13G	1G	‹1G	‹1G	‹1G	‹1G	120MG	0G	13MG	135MG

Easy Egg Strata

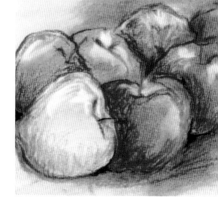

6 to 8 slices whole wheat bread, crusts trimmed	**1/2** cup skim milk
1 bunch green onions, chopped	**1/2** cup low-fat sour cream
1 pound extra-lean ham, chopped	**1/4** teaspoon nutmeg
1/2 large red bell pepper, chopped	Ground pepper to taste
12 Omega-3-enhanced eggs	**10** ounces reduced-fat Cheddar cheese, shredded

Line the bottom of a 9×13-inch baking pan or baking dish with the whole wheat bread slices. Sprinkle with the green onions, ham and bell pepper. Whisk the eggs, skim milk, sour cream, nutmeg and pepper in a bowl until blended.

Pour the egg mixture over the prepared layers and sprinkle with the cheese. Chill, covered, for 8 to 10 hours. Bake at 350 degrees for 30 to 40 minutes or until a knife inserted in the center comes out clean.

To increase your intake of Omega-3 fats, substitute Omega-3-enhanced eggs for regular eggs. They cook and taste the same as regular eggs.

NUTRIENTS PER SERVING

CAL	PROT	CARBO	T FAT	SAT. FAT	MONOUFA	FIBER	SOD	OMEGA-3 FATS	MG	K
251	23G	10G	13G	5G	3G	1G	582MG	‹1G	24MG	316MG

Wild Rice Quiche

2¹/₂	ounces frozen spinach, thawed and drained	1	tablespoon all-purpose flour
3	tablespoons dry whole wheat bread crumbs	¹/₃	cup 1% cottage cheese
1	tablespoon minced fresh parsley	¹/₄	cup (1 ounce) shredded reduced-fat Cheddar cheese
¹/₈	teaspoon pepper	1	(12-ounce) can evaporated skim milk
¹/₂	cup sliced mushrooms	³/₄	cup cooked wild rice
2	tablespoons chopped onion	3	Omega-3-enhanced eggs
¹/₄	teaspoon thyme	¹/₄	teaspoon salt
8	ounces spicy turkey sausage, crumbled, cooked and drained	¹/₈	teaspoon ground nutmeg
		¹/₈	teaspoon pepper

Squeeze the excess moisture from the spinach. Mix the bread crumbs, parsley and ¹/₈ teaspoon pepper in a bowl. Coat a 9-inch round baking dish with nonstick cooking spray and sprinkle the bread crumb mixture evenly over the bottom and side of the dish.

Spray a large skillet with nonstick cooking spray and heat over medium heat until hot. Add the mushrooms, onion and thyme and cook, covered, for 3 minutes or until the mushrooms are tender, stirring occasionally. Stir in the spinach and sausage and cook for 3 to 4 minutes or until most of the moisture evaporates, stirring frequently. Blend in the flour and cook for 1 minute, stirring frequently. Remove from the heat and stir in the cottage cheese and Cheddar cheese.

Mix the evaporated skim milk, wild rice, eggs, salt, nutmeg and ¹/₈ teaspoon pepper in a bowl. Stir in the sausage mixture and spoon into the prepared baking dish. Bake at 350 degrees for 35 minutes or until a knife inserted in the center comes out clean and the top is light brown. Cool on a wire rack for 5 minutes and cut into wedges.

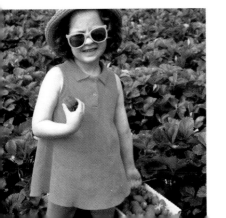

NUTRIENTS PER SERVING — Yield: 6 servings

CAL	PROT	CARBO	T FAT	SAT. FAT	MONOUFA	FIBER	SOD	OMEGA-3 FA	MG	K
212	21G	14G	7G	2G	2G	1G	518MG	<1G	46MG	452MG

Honey Wheat Bread

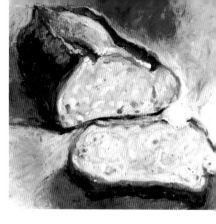

1½ teaspoons dry yeast	1¼ cups warm water
2 tablespoons warm water	1¾ cups all-purpose flour
3 tablespoons honey	1¼ cups whole wheat flour
1 tablespoon canola oil	1 cup ground flaxseed
½ teaspoon salt	

Dissolve the yeast in 2 tablespoons warm water in a bowl. Let stand for 5 minutes or until bubbly. Stir in the honey, canola oil, salt and 1¼ cups warm water. Add 1 cup of the all-purpose flour, the whole wheat flour and flaxseed and mix well. Stir in enough of the remaining all-purpose flour to make a soft and easily handled dough.

Turn the dough onto a lightly floured surface and knead for 10 minutes or until smooth and elastic. Shape into a loaf in a 5x9-inch loaf pan sprayed with nonstick cooking spray.

Let rise, covered, in a warm environment for 1 hour or until doubled in bulk. Bake at 350 degrees for 40 to 50 minutes or until the loaf is brown on top and sounds hollow when lightly tapped. Cool in the pan for 10 minutes. Remove to a wire rack to cool completely.

Grind flaxseed in a blender or coffee mill to the consistency of cornmeal for flaxseed meal. Generally, ⅔ cup of flaxseed yields 1 cup of flaxseed meal. Store the flaxseed meal in the refrigerator to preserve the highest amount of nutrients. Use within a few weeks.

NUTRIENTS PER SLICE   Yield: 10 slices

CAL	PROT	CARBO	T FAT	SAT. FAT	MONOUFA	FIBER	SOD	OMEGA-3 FATS	MG	K
228	7G	38G	6G	1G	2G	6G	122MG	3G	73MG	188MG

Nuts are a leading source of vitamin E and magnesium and also contain protein, fiber, potassium, calcium, phosphorus, and iron. Moreover, nuts contain phytochemicals—plant components that provide powerful protection against heart disease, stroke, and other chronic diseases.

Fruit and Nut Muffins

1¹/₂ cups all-purpose flour	2 apples, peeled and shredded
1 cup packed brown sugar	1 cup walnuts or soy nuts, ground
³/₄ cup ground flaxseed	¹/₂ cup raisins, dried cranberries or other dried fruit
³/₄ cup oat bran	
2 teaspoons baking soda	1 cup buttermilk
2 teaspoons ground cinnamon	2 Omega-3-enhanced eggs
1 teaspoon baking powder	2 tablespoons canola oil
¹/₂ teaspoon salt	1 teaspoon vanilla extract
1¹/₂ cups shredded carrots	

Combine the flour, brown sugar, flaxseed, oat bran, baking soda, cinnamon, baking powder and salt in a bowl and mix well. Stir in the carrots, apples, walnuts and raisins. Whisk the buttermilk, eggs, canola oil and vanilla in a bowl until blended. Add the buttermilk mixture to the flour mixture and stir just until moistened; the batter will be lumpy.

Fill nonstick muffin cups 2/3 full and bake at 350 degrees for 15 to 20 minutes or until the muffins test done. Remove the muffins to a wire rack to cool.

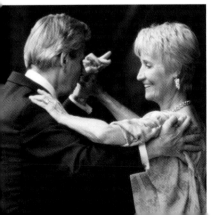

NUTRIENTS PER MUFFIN									Yield: 18 muffins	
CAL	PROT	CARBO	T FAT	SAT. FAT	MONOUFA	FIBER	SOD	OMEGA-3 FA	MG	K
206	5G	32G	8G	1G	2G	3G	267MG	2G	49MG	237MG

Raisin Muffins

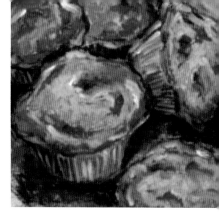

1¹/₄ cups whole wheat pastry flour

³/₄ cup ground flaxseed

¹/₂ cup sugar

1 teaspoon baking soda

¹/₂ teaspoon ground cinnamon

¹/₄ teaspoon ground nutmeg

¹/₄ teaspoon salt

1 cup buttermilk

¹/₂ cup unsweetened applesauce

2 Omega-3-enhanced eggs

2 tablespoons canola oil

¹/₂ cup golden raisins

Combine the whole wheat pastry flour, flaxseed, sugar, baking soda, cinnamon, nutmeg and salt in a bowl and mix well. Whisk the buttermilk, applesauce, eggs and canola oil in a bowl until combined and stir in the raisins. Add the buttermilk mixture to the flour mixture and mix just until moistened; do not overmix.

Spoon the batter into muffin cups sprayed with nonstick cooking spray or lined with paper liners. Bake at 375 degrees for 30 to 35 minutes or until the muffins test done. Remove the muffins to a wire rack to cool.

NUTRIENTS PER MUFFIN   Yield: 18 muffins

CAL	PROT	CARBO	T FAT	SAT. FAT	MONOUFA	FIBER	SOD	OMEGA-3 FATS	MG	K
121	3G	18G	4G	‹1G	2G	3G	127MG	1G	23MG	100MG

Spoon pancake batter into a sealable plastic bag. Snip off one corner and squeeze out silly shapes onto the hot griddle.

Brown Sugar and Cinnamon Pancakes

1 cup skim milk	**1/4** teaspoon salt
2/3 cup old-fashioned oats	**1/4** teaspoon ground cinnamon
2/3 cup all-purpose flour	**2** Omega-3-enhanced eggs, beaten
2 tablespoons brown sugar	**2** teaspoons canola oil
1¹/2 teaspoons baking powder	**1/4** teaspoon vanilla extract

Heat the skim milk in a small saucepan until hot. Remove from the heat and stir in the oats. Let stand, covered, for 5 minutes.

Combine the flour, brown sugar, baking powder, salt and cinnamon in a bowl and mix well. Make a well in the center of the flour mixture. Whisk the eggs, canola oil and vanilla in a bowl until blended. Pour the oat mixture and egg mixture into the well and stir just until moistened.

Pour 1/4 cup of the batter onto a hot griddle and cook for 4 minutes or until golden brown on both sides, turning once. Remove to a baking sheet and keep warm in a 200-degree oven. Repeat the process with the remaining batter.

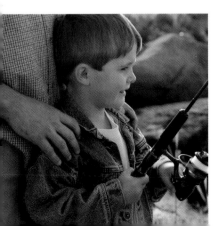

NUTRIENTS PER PANCAKE   Yield: 8 pancakes

CAL	PROT	CARBO	T FAT	SAT. FAT	MONOUFA	FIBER	SOD	OMEGA-3 FA	MG	K
122	5G	19G	3G	‹1G	1G	1G	196MG	‹1G	20MG	119MG

Banana Waffles

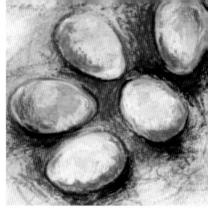

1   **cup skim milk**

1/3 **cup oat bran**

11/3 **cups mashed bananas**
     (2 medium bananas)

1   **cup skim milk**

1   **Omega-3-enhanced egg**

1   **tablespoon canola oil**

1   **cup all-purpose flour**

1/2 **cup whole wheat flour**

11/2 **teaspoons ground cinnamon**

3/4 **teaspoon baking powder**

Combine 1 cup skim milk and the oat bran in a medium microwave-safe bowl and mix well. Microwave on High for 2 minutes or until the mixture comes to a boil and stir.

Combine the bananas, 1 cup skim milk, the egg and canola oil in a blender and process at high speed until smooth. Add the hot oat bran mixture gradually, processing constantly until smooth.

Mix the all-purpose flour, whole wheat flour, cinnamon and baking powder in a bowl. Add the banana mixture to the flour mixture and stir just until the large lumps disappear. Pour about 1/2 cup of the batter onto a hot waffle iron and bake until the steam stops. Repeat the process with the remaining batter. Keep warm in a 200-degree oven.

NUTRIENTS PER WAFFLE   Yield: 12 (4-inch) waffles

CAL	PROT	CARBO	T FAT	SAT. FAT	MONOUFA	FIBER	SOD	OMEGA-3 FATS	MG	K
114	4G	21G	2G	‹1G	1G	2G	54MG	‹1G	27MG	205MG

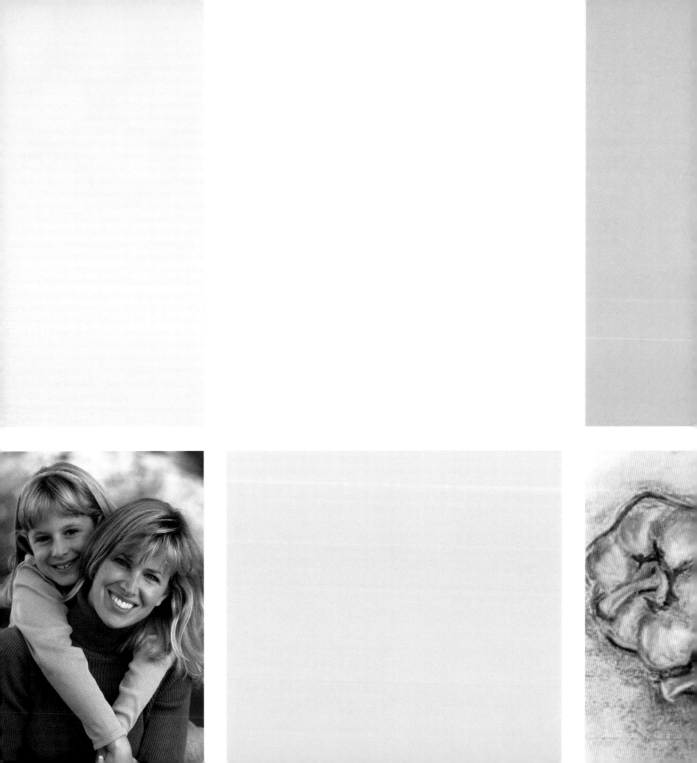

salads sides and sauces

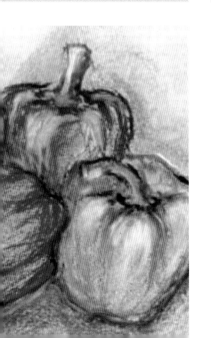

These dishes are colorful, flavorful, and healthy—the perfect complement to any meal. You will have no problem getting your daily veggies with these tasty sides. Vitamins and minerals never tasted so good.

Strawberry Orange Salad

By eating six grams of soluble fiber per day, you can achieve a modest lowering of your total cholesterol and LDL cholesterol.

2 **cups orange sections**	1/4 **teaspoon pepper**
11/2 **cups sliced fresh strawberries**	1/8 **teaspoon salt**
1 **tablespoon honey**	3 **cups torn fresh spinach**
1 **teaspoon extra-virgin olive oil**	1 **to 2 tablespoons honey-roasted soy nuts**
1/4 **teaspoon ground cinnamon**	

Combine the orange sections and strawberries in a salad bowl and mix gently. Whisk the honey, olive oil, cinnamon, pepper and salt in a bowl until blended and drizzle over the orange mixture, tossing gently to coat. Let stand for 30 minutes.

Add the spinach and soy nuts to the fruit mixture and mix gently. Serve immediately.

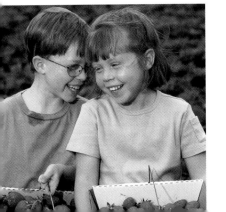

NUTRIENTS PER SERVING

Yield: 4 servings

CAL	PROT	CARBO	T FAT	SAT. FAT	MONOUFA	FIBER	SOD	OMEGA-3 FA	MG	K
112	3G	22G	2G	‹1G	1G	5G	105MG	‹1G	35MG	386MG

Asian Chicken Salad

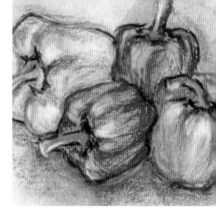

Asian Vinaigrette

1/2	cup rice wine vinegar or white vinegar
1/4	cup low-sodium soy sauce
3	tablespoons packed brown sugar
1	tablespoon dark sesame oil

Chicken Salad

1	head (1 1/4 pounds) napa cabbage, shredded
1/2	cup shredded red cabbage
1/2	cup julienned carrots
1	red bell pepper, chopped
2	green onions, chopped (white and green parts)
1	pound cooked boneless skinless chicken breasts, cut into strips
2	tablespoons flaxseed, toasted

For the vinaigrette, whisk the vinegar, soy sauce, brown sugar and sesame oil in a bowl until incorporated.

For the salad, toss the cabbage, carrots, bell pepper and green onions in a large salad bowl. Drizzle with the vinaigrette and top with the chicken. Sprinkle with the flaxseed and serve immediately.

NUTRIENTS PER SERVING   Yield: 6 servings

CAL	PROT	CARBO	T FAT	SAT. FAT	MONOUFA	FIBER	SOD	OMEGA-3 FATS	MG	K
232	26G	17G	6G	1G	1G	3G	485MG	1G	41MG	343MG

Salmon Salad **Monterey**

Lemon Dijon Dressing

- **3** tablespoons extra-virgin olive oil
- **1¹/₂** tablespoons lemon juice
- **1¹/₂** teaspoons finely chopped fresh chives
- **1** teaspoon honey
- **¹/₂** teaspoon Dijon mustard

Salmon Salad

- **1** (1¹/₄-pound) salmon fillet, skin removed
- **10** ounces dark green leafy lettuce, torn
- **1** cup red seedless grapes, cut into halves
- **¹/₃** cup walnuts, chopped

For the dressing, whisk the olive oil, lemon juice, chives, honey and Dijon mustard in a bowl until incorporated.

For the salad, cut the fillet into 4 equal portions and arrange in a single layer on a lightly oiled broiler rack in a broiler pan. Brush both sides of the fillets with some of the dressing. Broil 4 inches from the heat source for 7 to 9 minutes or until the fillets flake easily.

Toss the lettuce, grapes and walnuts in a bowl and spoon equal portions of the lettuce mixture on each of 4 serving plates. Arrange 1 fillet over the top of each salad and drizzle equally with the remaining dressing.

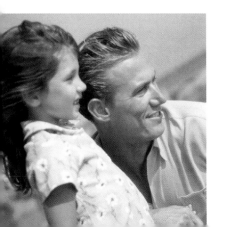

NUTRIENTS PER SERVING — Yield: 4 servings

CAL	PROT	CARBO	T FAT	SAT. FAT	MONOUFA	FIBER	SOD	OMEGA-3 FA	MG	K
450	35G	14G	29G	4G	15G	3G	120MG	2G	53MG	753MG

Roasted Broccoli Salad

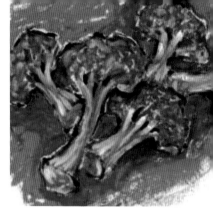

6	**Roma tomatoes, cut into halves**
1¹/₂	**teaspoons extra-virgin olive oil**
1	**bunch (1¹/₂ pounds) broccoli**
1¹/₂	**tablespoons extra-virgin olive oil**
2	**large garlic cloves, thinly sliced**
³/₄	**teaspoon coarse salt**

	Freshly ground pepper to taste
2	**tablespoons sliced almonds or pine nuts**
2	**bunches arugula, trimmed**
4	**teaspoons balsamic vinegar**

Toss the tomatoes with 1¹/₂ teaspoons olive oil in a bowl and set aside. Cut the broccoli into florets and trim the stalks of any tough portions. Peel the stalks and cut diagonally into ¹/₄-inch slices. Toss the broccoli florets and stalk slices with 1¹/₂ tablespoons olive oil in a bowl. Arrange the florets and sliced stalks on a baking sheet, leaving room for the tomatoes.

Roast at 450 degrees for 5 minutes. Arrange the tomatoes cut side up in a single layer on the baking sheet and sprinkle with the garlic, salt and pepper. Roast for 10 to 15 minutes longer or just until the vegetables are fork-tender.

Spread the almonds in a small skillet and toast over medium heat for 4 to 5 minutes or until golden brown. Remove to a plate to cool. Divide the arugula equally among 4 dinner plates. Top with equal portions of the roasted broccoli mixture and sprinkle with the almonds. Drizzle with the vinegar and serve hot.

> Microwave garlic cloves for fifteen seconds and the skins will slip right off.

NUTRIENTS PER SERVING　　　　　　　　**Yield: 6 servings**

CAL	PROT	CARBO	T FAT	SAT. FAT	MONOUFA	FIBER	SOD	OMEGA-3 FATS	MG	K
107	5G	11G	6G	1G	4G	5G	329MG	<1G	48MG	587MG

Plan your meals well to decrease your need for snacks.

Chinese Coleslaw

Olive Oil Vinaigrette

- **¹/₃ cup vinegar**
- **¹/₄ cup sugar**
- **¹/₈ teaspoon salt**
- **¹/₃ cup extra-virgin olive oil**

Coleslaw

- **1 (16-ounce) package shredded cabbage slaw**
- **4 green onions, chopped**
- **¹/₄ cup slivered almonds**
- **¹/₄ cup sunflower seed kernels**

For the vinaigrette, whisk the vinegar, sugar and salt in a bowl until blended. Add the olive oil gradually, whisking constantly until incorporated.

For the coleslaw, toss the cabbage slaw, green onions, almonds and sunflower seed kernels in a bowl. Add the vinaigrette and mix until coated.

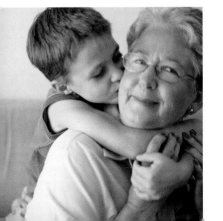

NUTRIENTS PER SERVING   Yield: 8 servings

CAL	PROT	CARBO	T FAT	SAT. FAT	MONOUFA	FIBER	SOD	OMEGA-3 FA	MG	K
175	3G	12G	14G	2G	8G	2G	52MG	‹1G	13MG	55MG

Cucumber Salad

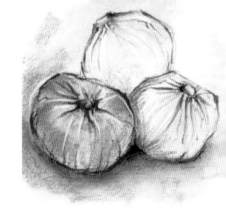

¹/₂ **cup low-fat sour cream**

¹/₂ **cup low-fat mayonnaise**

2 tablespoons plus 1 teaspoon red wine vinegar

2 tablespoons plus 1 teaspoon sugar

¹/₄ **teaspoon pepper**

¹/₈ **teaspoon salt**

3 cucumbers, sliced

1 onion, sliced

Combine the sour cream, mayonnaise, vinegar, sugar, pepper and salt in a bowl and mix well. Add the cucumbers and onion to the sour cream mixture and mix until coated. Chill, covered, for 1 to 2 hours before serving.

NUTRIENTS PER SERVING   Yield: 6 servings

CAL	PROT	CARBO	T FAT	SAT. FAT	MONOUFA	FIBER	SOD	OMEGA-3 FATS	MG	K
111	3G	16G	4G	2G	0G	2G	236MG	0G	2MG	335MG

Mediterranean Salad

1	cup chopped carrots	2	ounces feta cheese, crumbled
1	cup chopped broccoli	2	tablespoons extra-virgin olive oil
1	cup chopped cauliflower	1	tablespoon balsamic vinegar
1	cup chopped celery	1	teaspoon ground cumin
1/4	cup sliced kalamata olives		Salt and pepper to taste

Combine the carrots, broccoli, cauliflower, celery, olives and cheese in a bowl and mix well. Whisk the olive oil, vinegar, cumin, salt and pepper in a bowl.

Add the olive oil mixture to the carrot mixture and toss to coat. Serve with toasted pita points. You may substitute with your favorite vegetables if desired.

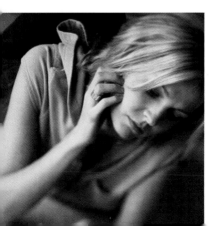

NUTRIENTS PER SERVING

Yield: 4 servings

CAL	PROT	CARBO	T FAT	SAT. FAT	MONOUFA	FIBER	SOD	OMEGA-3 FA	MG	K
145	4G	9G	11G	3G	7G	3G	292MG	<1G	19MG	340MG

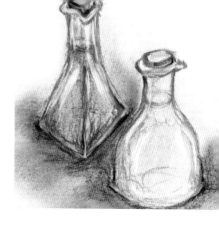

Balsamic Vinaigrette

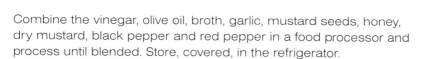

$1/2$ **cup plus 2 tablespoons balsamic vinegar**

1 **cup extra-virgin olive oil**

$1/4$ **cup low-sodium chicken broth or water**

5 **garlic cloves, minced**

$1^1/2$ **tablespoons mustard seeds**

$1^1/2$ **teaspoons honey**

$3/4$ **tablespoon dry mustard**

Black pepper to taste

Red pepper flakes to taste

Combine the vinegar, olive oil, broth, garlic, mustard seeds, honey, dry mustard, black pepper and red pepper in a food processor and process until blended. Store, covered, in the refrigerator.

You may mix in a jar with a tight-fitting lid. Drizzle over your favorite salad or use as a dipping sauce for crusty French bread.

The following are handy substitutions if ingredients are unavailable: substitute $1/8$ teaspoon garlic powder for 1 small garlic clove; substitute 3 or 4 slices of crumbled whole wheat bread for 1 cup dry bread crumbs; substitute a mixture of $2/3$ cup water and $1/3$ cup tomato paste for 1 cup tomato sauce; or substitute a mixture of $2^1/2$ cups water and 6 ounces tomato paste for 3 cups tomato juice.

NUTRIENTS PER 2 TABLESPOONS   Yield: 16 (2-tablespoon) servings

CAL	PROT	CARBO	T FAT	SAT. FAT	MONOUFA	FIBER	SOD	OMEGA-3 FATS	MG	K
148	<1G	5G	14G	2G	11G	<1G	17MG	<1G	3MG	18MG

Caesar Salad Dressing

2 cups nonfat plain yogurt	**2** tablespoons balsamic vinegar
1 cup (4 ounces) grated Parmesan cheese	**1** tablespoon Worcestershire sauce
	4 garlic cloves, minced
2 tablespoons lemon juice	**2** teaspoons anchovy paste

Combine the yogurt, 1 cup cheese, the lemon juice, balsamic vinegar, Worcestershire sauce, garlic and anchovy paste in a blender or food processor and process until smooth. Serve over torn romaine on salad plates. Garnish with croutons and additional freshly grated Parmesan cheese.

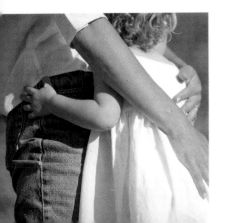

NUTRIENTS PER 2 TABLESPOONS								Yield: 18 (2-tablespoon) servings		
CAL	PROT	CARBO	T FAT	SAT. FAT	MONOUFA	FIBER	SOD	OMEGA-3 FA	MG	K
36	3G	4G	1G	1G	‹1G	‹1G	93MG	‹1G	2MG	19MG

Chicken Wild Rice Soup

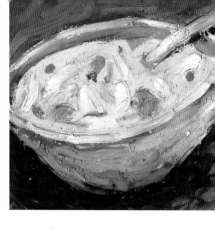

¹/₂   cup wild rice

2   cups water

1   tablespoon extra-virgin olive oil

4   (4-ounce) boneless skinless chicken breasts, cubed

1   onion, chopped

¹/₂   cup chopped celery

4   cups skim milk

¹/₄   cup all-purpose flour

2   teaspoons low-sodium chicken base

¹/₄   cup (¹/₂ stick) butter

1   (14-ounce) can sliced carrots, drained

3   tablespoons sliced almonds

3   tablespoons parsley flakes

1   tablespoon rosemary

1   teaspoon all-purpose seasoning

Soak the wild rice in 1 cup of the water in a bowl for 6 to 8 hours; drain. Bring the remaining 1 cup water to a boil in a saucepan and stir in the wild rice. Return to a boil and boil for 10 minutes or until the water level drops below the rice. Remove from the heat.

Heat the olive oil in a medium saucepan over medium heat. Add the chicken, onion and celery and cook for 10 to 15 minutes or until brown and slightly crisp, stirring frequently. Whisk the skim milk, flour and chicken base in a large saucepan until blended. Stir in the chicken mixture, butter, carrots, almonds, parsley flakes, rosemary and all-purpose seasoning. Bring to a boil and reduce the heat to low.

Add the wild rice to the soup mixture and simmer for 15 minutes, stirring occasionally and adding additional water if needed for a thinner consistency. Ladle into soup bowls and serve immediately.

Under the weather? Sipping hot soup and breathing in the steam clears congestion. Spices such as garlic and pepper also thin mucus and ease breathing.

NUTRIENTS PER SERVING   Yield: 8 servings

CAL	PROT	CARBO	T FAT	SAT. FAT	MONOUFA	FIBER	SOD	OMEGA-3 FATS	MG	K
260	19G	23G	10G	4G	4G	3G	381MG	<1G	53MG	406MG

Make your own **White Sauce** by heating 2 tablespoons unsalted butter in a saucepan. Stir in 2 tablespoons all-purpose flour and cook until bubbly. Gradually add 1 cup skim milk and cook until thickened, stirring constantly. Add the desired amount of reduced-fat cheese for a great **Cheese Sauce** and cook until blended.

Asparagus with Mustard Sauce

4	pounds fresh asparagus spears	2	tablespoons lemon juice
4	quarts water	1/4	teaspoon salt
2	tablespoons Dijon mustard	1	tablespoon mustard seeds

Snap off the thick woody ends of the asparagus spears and discard. Bring the water to a boil in an 8-quart stockpot and add 1/2 of the asparagus spears. Cook for 3 minutes and immediately plunge the asparagus into a bowl of ice water to stop the cooking process and preserve the bright green color. Drain and pat dry with paper towels. Repeat the process with the remaining asparagus.

Combine the Dijon mustard, lemon juice and salt in a bowl and mix well. Heat a large nonstick skillet over medium heat and add the mustard seeds. Cook for 1 minute, stirring constantly. Add the asparagus and Dijon mustard mixture to the hot skillet and cook for 2 minutes or until heated through, stirring frequently. Serve immediately.

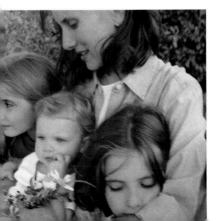

NUTRIENTS PER SERVING Yield: 8 servings

CAL	PROT	CARBO	T FAT	SAT. FAT	MONOUFA	FIBER	SOD	OMEGA-3 FA	MG	K
57	6G	10G	1G	‹1G	‹1G	5G	172MG	‹1G	36MG	478MG

Lemon Dijon Asparagus

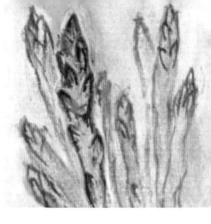

1¹/₂ **pounds fresh asparagus spears**	1 **tablespoon minced fresh chives**
2 **tablespoons lemon juice**	2 **teaspoons minced lemon zest**
1 **tablespoon extra-virgin olive oil**	1 **teaspoon sugar**
1 **tablespoon Dijon mustard**	¹/₄ **teaspoon freshly ground pepper**
1 **tablespoon minced fresh parsley**	

Snap off the thick woody ends of the asparagus spears and discard. Blanch the asparagus spears in boiling water in a saucepan for 3 minutes. Immediately plunge the spears into a bowl of ice water to stop the cooking process and preserve the bright green color. Drain and pat dry with paper towels. Arrange the asparagus on a serving platter.

Whisk the lemon juice, olive oil, Dijon mustard, parsley, chives, lemon zest, sugar and pepper in a bowl until combined. Drizzle the Dijon mustard mixture over the asparagus and serve at room temperature.

NUTRIENTS PER SERVING   Yield: 4 servings

CAL	PROT	CARBO	T FAT	SAT. FAT	MONOUFA	FIBER	SOD	OMEGA-3 FATS	MG	K
77	4G	9G	4G	1G	3G	4G	99MG	‹1G	25MG	369MG

Green Beans Amandine

2	**tablespoons extra-virgin olive oil**	**2**	**tablespoons water**
1¹/₂	**pounds fresh green beans, trimmed**	**1**	**tablespoon cornstarch**
1¹/₂	**cups low-sodium chicken broth**	**1**	**tablespoon lemon juice**
¹/₄	**teaspoon freshly ground pepper**	**¹/₄**	**cup sliced almonds, toasted**
	Salt to taste		

Heat the olive oil in a large skillet over medium-high heat and add the beans. Sauté for 5 minutes. Stir in the broth, pepper and salt and bring to a boil. Reduce the heat and simmer, covered, for 15 minutes, stirring occasionally.

Mix the water and cornstarch in a small bowl and add to the bean mixture. Return to a boil and boil for 1 minute, stirring constantly. Stir in the lemon juice. Spoon the beans into a serving bowl and sprinkle with the almonds just before serving.

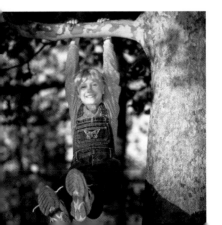

NUTRIENTS PER ¹/₂ CUP								Yield: 8 (¹/₂-cup) servings		
CAL	PROT	CARBO	T FAT	SAT. FAT	MONOUFA	FIBER	SOD	OMEGA-3 FA	MG	K
88	3G	8G	6G	1G	4G	3G	20MG	‹1G	31MG	241MG

Southwest Corn Skillet

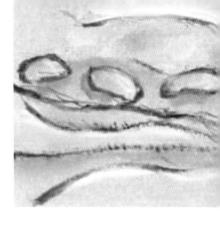

1	**red bell pepper, chopped**
1	**tablespoon finely chopped jalapeño chile**
1	**tablespoon butter or trans-fat-free margarine**
1½	**teaspoons ground cumin**
1	**(16-ounce) package frozen corn, thawed**

Sauté the bell pepper and jalapeño chile in the butter in a nonstick skillet until tender. Stir in the cumin and sauté for 30 seconds. Mix in the corn and sauté for 2 minutes longer or until heated through. Spoon into a serving bowl.

For a speedy side dish, combine chopped fresh tomatoes with basil, garlic powder, and a splash of extra-virgin olive oil. Toss the tomato mixture with hot cooked pasta and sprinkle with freshly grated Parmesan cheese. Serve immediately.

NUTRIENTS PER SERVING   Yield: 4 servings

CAL	PROT	CARBO	T FAT	SAT. FAT	MONOUFA	FIBER	SOD	OMEGA-3 FATS	MG	K
133	4G	25G	4G	2G	1G	3G	24MG	‹1G	24MG	302MG

Glazed Squash

Increase your water intake as you add fiber to your diet.

1	(1 1/2-pound) acorn squash	1/4	teaspoon salt
2	tablespoons maple syrup	1/8	teaspoon ground nutmeg
2	teaspoons butter or trans-fat-free margarine, melted		

Cut the squash crosswise into four 1-inch-thick slices and discard the seeds. Arrange the squash slices on a microwave-safe plate. Cover with plastic wrap and vent. Microwave on High for 6 minutes or until tender. Arrange the slices in a single layer on a baking sheet.

Combine the syrup, butter, salt and nutmeg in a bowl and mix well. Brush the squash with some of the syrup mixture and broil for 3 minutes or until bubbly. Drizzle with the remaining syrup mixture and serve immediately.

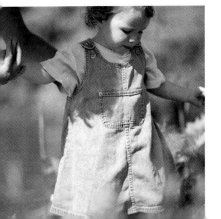

NUTRIENTS PER SERVING Yield: 2 servings

CAL	PROT	CARBO	T FAT	SAT. FAT	MONOUFA	FIBER	SOD	OMEGA-3 FA	MG	K
222	3G	49G	4G	2G	1G	5G	330MG	‹1G	112MG	1222MG

Honeyed Mashed Sweet Potatoes

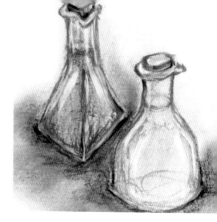

2   **pounds sweet potatoes**

1/2   **cup low-fat sour cream**

1/4   **cup honey**

   Ground nutmeg to taste

2   **tablespoons butter or trans-fat-free margarine, softened**

1   **tablespoon honey**

Peel the sweet potatoes and cut into 1-inch chunks. Arrange the sweet potato chunks in a single layer on a baking sheet and spray with olive oil nonstick cooking spray. Bake at 375 degrees for 45 minutes or until tender, turning occasionally.

Combine the sweet potatoes, sour cream, 1/4 cup honey, nutmeg and butter in a mixing bowl and beat at medium speed until smooth, scraping the bowl occasionally. Spoon the sweet potatoes into a serving bowl and drizzle with 1 tablespoon honey. Serve immediately.

NUTRIENTS PER SERVING   Yield: 8 servings

CAL	PROT	CARBO	T FAT	SAT. FAT	MONOUFA	FIBER	SOD	OMEGA-3 FATS	MG	K
199	3G	41G	4G	3G	1G	4G	70MG	<1G	<1MG	348MG

sides

Sweet Potato Strips

**1¹/2 pounds sweet potatoes
(about 3 medium)**

1 teaspoon salt

¹/4 teaspoon pepper

Cut the unpeeled sweet potatoes into 3-inch strips, approximately ¹/8 inch thick. Pat dry with paper towels and spray with nonstick cooking spray.

Arrange the strips in a single layer on a baking sheet and bake at 350 degrees for 20 to 30 minutes or until golden brown. Sprinkle with the salt and pepper and serve warm with Curried Mayonnaise Dip on page 28.

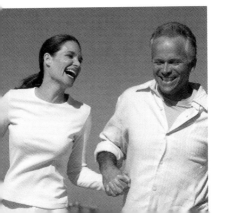

NUTRIENTS PER SERVING   Yield: 6 servings

CAL	PROT	CARBO	T FAT	SAT. FAT	MONOUFA	FIBER	SOD	OMEGA-3 FA	MG	K
65	1G	17G	0G	0G	0G	2G	410MG	0G	<1MG	175MG

Nutritional profile does not include the Curried Mayonnaise Dip.

Vegetables au Gratin

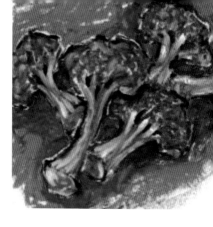

2	tablespoons extra-virgin olive oil	3	sweet potatoes, peeled and thinly sliced
1	tablespoon unsalted butter or trans-fat-free margarine		Salt and pepper to taste
1	onion, chopped	1	tablespoon unsalted butter or trans-fat-free margarine
1	cup sliced fresh mushrooms	2	cups skim milk
1	large carrot, thinly sliced	3	Omega-3-enhanced eggs
1	zucchini, thinly sliced	3	cups whole wheat bread crumbs
1	head broccoli, thinly sliced	1/4	cup (1 ounce) grated Parmesan cheese
1	head cauliflower, thinly sliced		
2 1/2	cups (10 ounces) shredded reduced-fat Cheddar cheese		

Heat the olive oil and 1 tablespoon butter in a skillet and add the onion. Sauté until light brown and stir in the mushrooms. Sauté for 2 minutes longer and remove from the heat. Layer 1/2 of the onion mixture, 1/2 of the carrot, 1/2 of the zucchini, 1/2 of the broccoli and 1/2 of the cauliflower in a 9x13-inch baking pan sprayed with nonstick cooking spray. Sprinkle with 1/3 of the Cheddar cheese and layer with the remaining onion mixture, remaining carrot, remaining zucchini, remaining broccoli and remaining cauliflower. Sprinkle with 1/2 of the remaining Cheddar cheese, layer with the sweet potatoes and sprinkle with salt and pepper. Dot with 1 tablespoon butter.

Whisk the skim milk and eggs in a bowl until blended and pour over the prepared layers. Bake, covered with foil, at 375 degrees for 30 minutes. Remove the foil and bake for 15 minutes. Sprinkle with the remaining Cheddar cheese, bread crumbs and Parmesan cheese and bake for 15 minutes longer. You may substitute any combination of your favorite vegetables for the ones mentioned.

NUTRIENTS PER SERVING   Yield: 8 servings

CAL	PROT	CARBO	T FAT	SAT. FAT	MONOUFA	FIBER	SOD	OMEGA-3 FATS	MG	K
349	20G	34G	17G	8G	5G	6G	245MG	<1G	42MG	697MG

Broccoli Tomato
Pasta Toss

12	**ounces mostaccioli or other pasta**	**¹/₈**	**teaspoon red pepper flakes**
2	**tablespoons extra-virgin olive oil**	**3**	**cups chopped fresh broccoli**
2	**tablespoons minced garlic**	**2**	**cups chopped fresh tomatoes or cherry tomato halves**
¹/₂	**cup white wine**		

Cook the pasta in boiling water in a 3- or 4-quart saucepan for 12 to 14 minutes or until al dente. Drain and return the pasta to the saucepan. Cover to keep warm.

Heat the olive oil in a large skillet over medium heat until hot. Add the garlic to the hot oil and sauté for 5 minutes. Reduce the heat to low and stir in the wine and red pepper flakes. Simmer until the mixture bubbles, stirring frequently. Stir in the broccoli.

Steam, covered, for 4 minutes or until the broccoli is bright green but still crunchy. Stir in the tomatoes and cook until heated through, stirring frequently. Remove from the heat and add the pasta, tossing until combined. Serve with freshly grated Parmesan cheese.

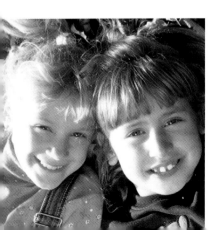

NUTRIENTS PER SERVING   **Yield: 6 servings**

CAL	PROT	CARBO	T FAT	SAT. FAT	MONOUFA	FIBER	SOD	OMEGA-3 FA	MG	K
294	10G	49G	6G	1G	4G	4G	19MG	‹1G	50MG	383MG

Pesto Vegetable Pasta

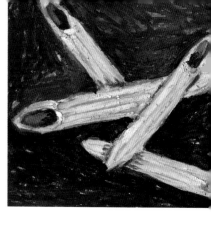

8 ounces pasta shells	**1/4** cup (1 ounce) grated Parmesan cheese
8 ounces fresh green beans, cut into 1-inch pieces	**3** tablespoons low-fat mayonnaise
2 carrots, julienned	**2** tablespoons coarsely chopped walnuts
1 yellow squash, thinly sliced	**3** garlic cloves, minced
1/2 cup fresh basil leaves	
1/2 cup plain nonfat yogurt	

Cook the pasta in boiling water in a saucepan for 7 minutes. Add the green beans and carrots to the saucepan and cook for 3 minutes longer or until the pasta is tender; drain. Combine the pasta mixture with the squash in a bowl and let stand until cool.

Combine the basil, yogurt, cheese, mayonnaise, walnuts and garlic in a food processor and process until puréed. Add the basil mixture to the pasta mixture and toss until coated. Serve at room temperature or chilled.

When using spaghetti, keep in mind that eight ounces uncooked pasta makes four cups cooked.

NUTRIENTS PER SERVING

Yield: 4 servings

CAL	PROT	CARBO	T FAT	SAT. FAT	MONOUFA	FIBER	SOD	OMEGA-3 FATS	MG	K
367	16G	62G	7G	2G	1G	10G	226MG	<1G	62MG	468MG

Tomato Alfredo Linguini

2	teaspoons extra-virgin olive oil	2	cups skim milk
2	garlic cloves, minced	1	cup (4 ounces) shredded reduced-fat Swiss cheese
2	(14-ounce) cans Italian-style diced tomatoes	1/2	cup dry white wine
1	tablespoon chopped fresh basil	1/2	teaspoon pepper
1/4	teaspoon pepper	1/4	teaspoon salt
1/4	teaspoon salt	8	cups hot cooked linguini (about 16 ounces uncooked linguini)
4	cups sliced fresh mushrooms	1/4	cup (1 ounce) freshly grated Parmesan cheese
1/2	cup all-purpose flour		

Heat the olive oil in a nonstick skillet over medium heat and add the garlic. Sauté for 30 seconds and stir in the undrained tomatoes, basil, 1/4 teaspoon pepper and 1/4 teaspoon salt. Reduce the heat to low and cook for 20 minutes or until of a sauce consistency, stirring occasionally. Coat a large saucepan with nonstick cooking spray and heat over medium-high heat. Add the mushrooms to the hot saucepan and cook for 5 minutes, stirring frequently. Remove the mushrooms to a bowl using a slotted spoon, reserving the pan juices. Mix the flour with the reserved pan juices. Add the skim milk gradually, whisking constantly until blended.

Cook over medium heat for 3 minutes or until thickened, stirring constantly. Stir in the Swiss cheese, wine, 1/2 teaspoon pepper and 1/4 teaspoon salt. Cook for 1 minute or until the cheese melts, stirring constantly. Remove from the heat and stir in the mushrooms. Toss the pasta and mushroom mixture in a large bowl and spoon into a 9x13-inch baking dish sprayed with nonstick cooking spray. Spread the tomato sauce over the prepared layer and sprinkle with the Parmesan cheese. Bake, covered, at 350 degrees for 20 minutes. Remove the cover and bake for 5 minutes longer.

NUTRIENTS PER SERVING · Yield: 8 servings

CAL	PROT	CARBO	T FAT	SAT. FAT	MONOUFA	FIBER	SOD	OMEGA-3 FA	MG	K
383	18G	62G	6G	3G	1G	3G	644MG	<1G	45MG	355MG

Freeze tomatoes in sealable freezer bags when plentiful. When ready for use in soups or sauces, simply run warm water into the bag. The skins can be removed with minimal peeling.

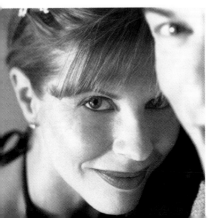

Toasted Walnut Pasta

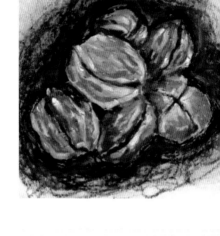

16	ounces penne or rigatoni	1/4	cup walnuts, coarsely chopped
1	cup packed fresh basil leaves	2	tablespoons coarsely chopped kalamata olives
1	garlic clove, minced		
1/4	cup low-sodium chicken broth	1	tablespoon grated Parmesan cheese
2	tablespoons extra-virgin olive oil		

Cook the pasta using package directions. Drain, reserving 1/4 cup of the cooking liquid. Cover the pasta to keep warm. Combine the basil and garlic in a food processor and process until finely chopped. Add the broth and olive oil gradually, processing constantly until incorporated.

Toast the walnuts in a large skillet over medium heat until light brown, stirring constantly. Toss the pasta with the basil mixture and reserved liquid in a bowl. Stir in the walnuts, olives and cheese and serve immediately.

NUTRIENTS PER SERVING   Yield: 6 servings

CAL	PROT	CARBO	T FAT	SAT. FAT	MONOUFA	FIBER	SOD	OMEGA-3 FATS	MG	K
417	17G	67G	10G	1G	4G	11G	53MG	<1G	48MG	139MG

Use the quick-soak method for dried beans to save time. Bring 1 pound of dried beans and 6 cups of water to a rolling boil in a large saucepan. Boil for 2 minutes. Remove from the heat and let stand, covered, for 1 hour; drain. Cook the beans as directed on the package. One cup of dried beans equals 2 to 3 cups of cooked beans.

Mushroom and Almond Pilaf

1	**quart chicken stock or canned low-sodium chicken broth**
	2 1/2 cups bulgur
	3 tablespoons extra-virgin olive oil

Salt and pepper to taste

12 ounces mushrooms

1/2 cup slivered almonds, toasted

2 tablespoons extra-virgin olive oil

Bring the stock to a boil in a large saucepan over high heat. Gradually add the bulgur to the hot stock; do not stir. Reduce the heat to low and simmer, covered, for 45 minutes or just until tender.

Heat 3 tablespoons olive oil in a saucepan until almost smoking. Immediately pour the hot oil over the cooked bulgur. Simmer, covered, for 7 minutes or until the bulgur is dry and tender. Season to taste with salt and pepper.

Heat 2 tablespoons olive oil in a medium skillet and stir in the mushrooms. Sauté for 4 minutes or until light brown. Stir the mushrooms and almonds into the bulgur and serve immediately.

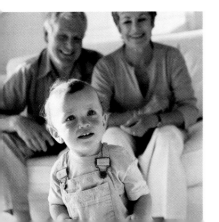

NUTRIENTS PER SERVING   Yield: 8 servings

CAL	PROT	CARBO	T FAT	SAT. FAT	MONOUFA	FIBER	SOD	OMEGA-3 FA	MG	K
321	11G	40G	14G	2G	10G	9G	179MG	<1G	95MG	506MG

Quinoa Pilaf

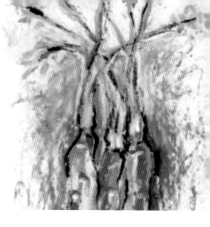

1/2	cup quinoa	1	bay leaf
1/2	onion, chopped	1	tablespoon grated lemon zest
2	carrots, chopped	1	tablespoon lemon juice
1	rib celery, chopped	1/2	cup frozen peas, thawed
1	tablespoon extra-virgin olive oil		Freshly ground pepper to taste
1	cup low-sodium chicken or vegetable broth, heated		

Rinse the quinoa with cold water and drain. Sauté the onion, carrots and celery in the olive oil in a saucepan until the vegetables are tender. Stir in the quinoa and cook for 1 minute, stirring constantly. Add the broth, bay leaf, lemon zest and lemon juice and mix well. Bring to a boil and reduce the heat.

Simmer, covered, for 15 to 20 minutes or until the liquid is absorbed and the quinoa is tender. Discard the bay leaf and stir in the peas. Season to taste with pepper.

NUTRIENTS PER SERVING — Yield: 4 servings

CAL	PROT	CARBO	T FAT	SAT. FAT	MONOUFA	FIBER	SOD	OMEGA-3 FATS	MG	K
156	5G	23G	5G	1G	3G	3G	72MG	1G	56MG	386MG

Corn Bread Stuffing

8	**ounces reduced-fat turkey sausage**	**2**	**apples, chopped**
2	**tablespoons apple juice**	**1/4**	**cup chopped fresh parsley**
1	**(16-ounce) package corn bread stuffing**	**1**	**tablespoon poultry seasoning**
1	**large onion, chopped**	**1/2**	**teaspoon ground thyme**
2	**ribs celery, chopped**	**1/2**	**teaspoon pepper**
1	**tablespoon unsalted butter or trans-fat-free margarine**	**1**	**cup low-sodium chicken broth**

Coat a large skillet with nonstick cooking spray and heat over medium heat. Add the sausage to the hot skillet and cook until brown and crumbly, stirring frequently; drain. Add the apple juice to the skillet and simmer until the juice evaporates, stirring constantly. Combine the sausage mixture with the stuffing crumbs in a bowl and mix well.

Sauté the onion and celery in the butter in a skillet until the onion is tender. Add the onion mixture, apples, parsley, poultry seasoning, thyme and pepper to the sausage mixture and mix well. Add the broth until the desired consistency and mix well.

Spoon the sausage mixture into a baking dish and cover with foil. Bake at 350 degrees for 30 minutes and remove the foil. Bake for 15 minutes longer or until golden brown. Use as the stuffing for the Stuffed Turkey Breast on page 100.

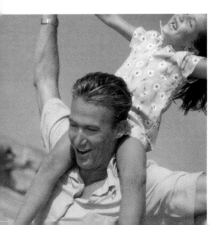

NUTRIENTS PER SERVING										Yield: 8 (3/4-cup) servings
CAL	PROT	CARBO	T FAT	SAT. FAT	MONOUFA	FIBER	SOD	OMEGA-3 FA	MG	K
296	9G	53G	6G	2G	2G	10G	829MG	<1G	35MG	278MG

Teriyaki Marinade

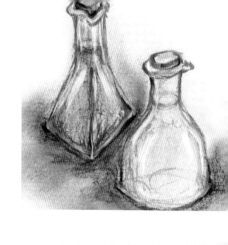

1	cup unsweetened pineapple juice	4	green onions, minced
3/4	cup low-sodium soy sauce	8	garlic cloves, minced
2/3	cup dry sherry	1	tablespoon sesame oil
1/4	cup packed brown sugar	1/4	teaspoon minced fresh ginger

Combine the pineapple juice, soy sauce, sherry, brown sugar, green onions, garlic, sesame oil and ginger in a jar with a tight-fitting lid and seal tightly. Shake to mix. Store in the refrigerator. This recipe provides enough marinade for 4 pounds of chicken, beef or fish.

NUTRIENTS PER 1/4 CUP   Yield: 12 (1/4-cup) servings

CAL	PROT	CARBO	T FAT	SAT. FAT	MONOUFA	FIBER	SOD	OMEGA-3 FATS	MG	K
63	1G	10G	1G	‹1G	0G	‹1G	609MG	0G	7MG	77MG

Cranberry Port Sauce

1	(12-ounce) package fresh cranberries	2	cinnamon sticks
1	cup sugar	2	tablespoons lemon juice
1	cup port	1	teaspoon grated lemon zest
		1/16	teaspoon ground cloves

Combine the cranberries, sugar, wine, cinnamon sticks, lemon juice, lemon zest and cloves in a medium saucepan and mix well. Simmer for 15 to 20 minutes or until the cranberries burst and the mixture thickens, stirring occasionally.

Discard the cinnamon sticks and store, covered, in the refrigerator. Serve with poultry or pork. You may substitute artificial sweetener for the sugar.

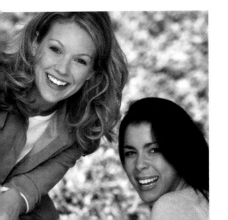

NUTRIENTS PER SERVING   Yield: 24 servings

CAL	PROT	CARBO	T FAT	SAT. FAT	MONOUFA	FIBER	SOD	OMEGA-3 FA	MG	K
55	<1G	12G	<1G	0G	0G	1G	1MG	0G	2MG	23MG

Honey Herb Sauce

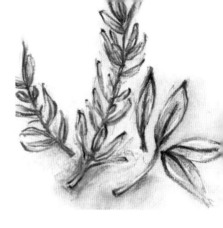

1/4 cup honey

2 tablespoons minced onion

2 tablespoons butter or trans-fat-free margarine

1/2 teaspoon thyme, crushed

Salt and pepper to taste

Combine the honey, onion, butter, thyme, salt and pepper in a small saucepan and bring to a boil, stirring occasionally. Cook for 2 minutes, stirring occasionally.

Toss the sauce with peas, zucchini, spinach, broccoli, green beans or vegetable of choice. Or, serve over hot cooked couscous as a vegetarian entrée or alone as a side dish.

Mealtime provides an arena to promote positive family connections and to develop a child's social awareness. Take this time to set good examples about nutrition.

NUTRIENTS PER SERVING   Yield: 6 servings

CAL	PROT	CARBO	T FAT	SAT. FAT	MONOUFA	FIBER	SOD	OMEGA-3 FATS	MG	K
78	<1G	12G	4G	2G	1G	<1G	28MG	<1G	1MG	13MG

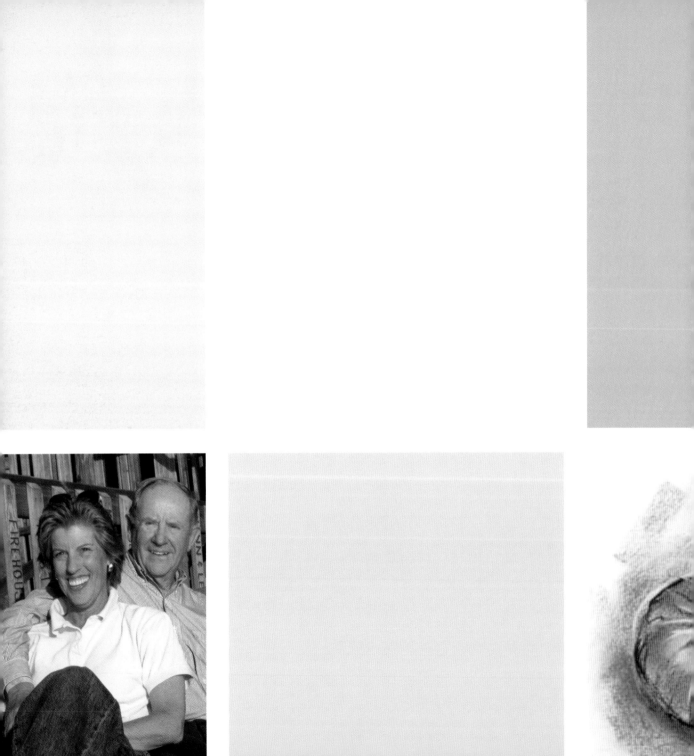

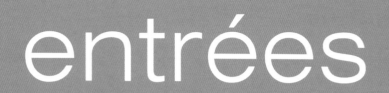

entrées

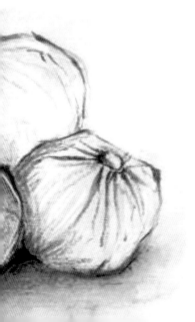

Whether you are cooking for one or hosting a dinner party, these delicious dishes are sure to please. Treat your heart to salmon and other healthy fish, as well as new twists on pork, beef, chicken, and beans.

Easy Beef Tenderloin with Wine Gravy

Beef Tenderloin

2	teaspoons minced fresh garlic
1	teaspoon salt
1	teaspoon chopped fresh thyme, or 1/2 teaspoon dried thyme
1/2	teaspoon freshly ground pepper
2	pounds beef tenderloin
1	tablespoon olive oil

Wine Gravy

1	cup low-sodium beef broth
1/2	cup red wine
	Freshly ground pepper to taste

For the tenderloin, preheat the oven to 500 degrees. Mix the garlic, salt, thyme and pepper in a small bowl. Brush the tenderloin with the olive oil and rub the garlic mixture over the surface. Arrange the tenderloin in a roasting pan and place on the middle oven rack. Immediately reduce the oven temperature to 400 degrees.

Roast for 30 minutes or until a meat thermometer registers 145 degrees for medium-rare. Remove the tenderloin to a platter and drape with foil, reserving the pan drippings. Let stand for 10 minutes before carving.

For the gravy, heat the reserved pan drippings, broth and wine in a saucepan until the desired consistency, stirring frequently. Season to taste with pepper and serve with the tenderloin.

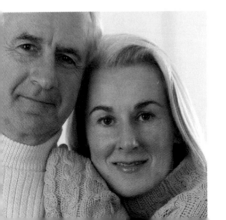

NUTRIENTS PER SERVING   Yield: 8 servings

CAL	PROT	CARBO	T FAT	SAT. FAT	MONOUFA	FIBER	SOD	OMEGA-3 FA	MG	K
196	25G	1G	9G	3G	4G	<1G	350MG	<1G	23MG	348MG

Beef and Mushroom Pilaf

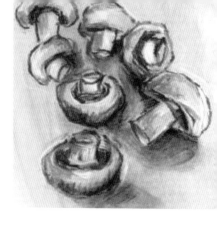

1	pound boneless beef sirloin	1	(14-ounce) can low-sodium beef broth	
4	teaspoons extra-virgin olive oil	1	tablespoon Worcestershire sauce	
3	cups fresh mushrooms, sliced	1	cup chopped red bell pepper	
2	garlic cloves, minced	1/2	teaspoon sesame oil	
1	cup basmati rice or long grain rice	1/2	cup sliced green onions	
			Low-sodium soy sauce (optional)	

Cut the beef into 3-inch-long strips. Heat the olive oil in a 10-inch skillet over medium-high heat and add the beef. Cook until brown on both sides, turning occasionally. Remove the beef to a platter using a slotted spoon, reserving the pan drippings.

Cook the mushrooms and garlic in the reserved pan drippings for 3 minutes or until the mushrooms begin to brown, stirring frequently. Stir in the rice, broth, Worcestershire sauce, bell pepper and sesame oil and bring to a boil. Stir in the beef and reduce the heat to low.

Simmer, covered, for 15 to 20 minutes or until the rice is tender and the liquid is absorbed; do not stir. Garnish with the green onions and serve with soy sauce.

Beef from grass-fed cattle typically has one-half the saturated fat of grain-fed beef. Besides being lower in saturated fats, grass-fed beef is higher in Omega-3 fatty acids, vitamin E, and conjugated linoleic acid, another beneficial fatty acid. If you eat beef regularly and have heart disease, the switch to grass-fed beef is a good nutritional choice.

NUTRIENTS PER SERVING   Yield: 4 servings

CAL	PROT	CARBO	T FAT	SAT. FAT	MONOUFA	FIBER	SOD	OMEGA-3 FATS	MG	K
325	31G	26G	11G	3G	6G	2G	129MG	‹1G	37MG	820MG

Szechwan Beef Stir-Fry

1	(1-pound) beef flank steak, trimmed	2	garlic cloves, crushed
2	tablespoons low-sodium soy sauce	1	tablespoon minced fresh ginger
1	tablespoon sesame oil	1/4	teaspoon red pepper flakes
1 1/2	teaspoons sugar	1	small red bell pepper, cut into 1-inch pieces
1	teaspoon cornstarch	1	(8-ounce) can whole baby corn, drained
1	tablespoon sesame oil	4	ounces snow peas, julienned

Freeze the steak for 30 minutes or until firm. Cut the steak lengthwise into 2 equal portions and cut each portion across the grain into 1/8-inch strips. Combine the soy sauce, 1 tablespoon sesame oil, the sugar and cornstarch in a bowl and mix until blended. Pour over the beef in a shallow dish, turning to coat.

Heat 1 tablespoon sesame oil in a wok or large nonstick skillet over medium-high heat. Add the garlic, ginger and red pepper flakes to the hot oil and stir-fry for 30 seconds. Add the bell pepper and corn and stir-fry for 1 1/2 minutes. Mix in the snow peas and stir-fry for 30 seconds. Remove the vegetable mixture to a bowl using a slotted spoon, reserving the pan drippings.

Stir-fry the beef 1/2 at a time in the reserved pan drippings for 2 to 3 minutes. Return the vegetable mixture to the wok and stir-fry just until heated through. Serve immediately.

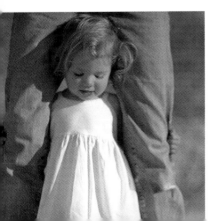

NUTRIENTS PER SERVING   Yield: 4 servings

CAL	PROT	CARBO	T FAT	SAT. FAT	MONOUFA	FIBER	SOD	OMEGA-3 FA	MG	K
262	25G	8G	14G	4G	5G	2G	355MG	‹1G	29MG	382MG

Fiesta Chili

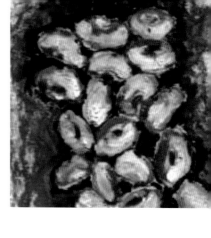

1   pound extra-lean ground beef or soy crumbles

1   cup chopped onion

1   cup chopped green bell pepper

2   (14-ounce) cans diced tomatoes

2   (15-ounce) cans black beans, drained

1¹/₂ cups low-sodium beef broth

1   tablespoon chili powder

3   garlic cloves, crushed

1¹/₂ teaspoons ground cumin

³/₄ teaspoon oregano

¹/₈ teaspoon pepper

     Low-fat sour cream (optional)

     Chopped fresh cilantro

Brown the ground beef with the onion and bell pepper in a stockpot, stirring until the ground beef is crumbly; drain. Add the undrained tomatoes, beans, broth, chili powder, garlic, cumin, oregano and pepper and mix well. Bring to a boil and reduce the heat to low, stirring occasionally.

Simmer for 15 minutes or until slightly thickened, stirring occasionally. Ladle into chili bowls and garnish with sour cream and chopped cilantro. Serve immediately.

Replace the ground beef in your chili and other casseroles with extra beans or soy crumbles. Experiment with different varieties of beans.

NUTRIENTS PER SERVING   Yield: 6 servings

CAL	PROT	CARBO	T FAT	SAT. FAT	MONOUFA	FIBER	SOD	OMEGA-3 FATS	MG	K
281	27G	34G	6G	2G	‹1G	11G	749MG	‹1G	8MG	164MG

Honey Mustard Tenderloin

Add water to the bottom of a broiler pan before baking. The water will absorb the smoke and grease and make the food more tender.

1/4	cup honey	1	tablespoon Dijon mustard
2	tablespoons vinegar	1/2	teaspoon paprika
2	tablespoons brown sugar	1	(3-pound) pork tenderloin

Combine the honey, vinegar, brown sugar, Dijon mustard and paprika in a bowl and mix well. Coat the tenderloin with the honey mixture and arrange in a roasting pan.

Roast at 375 degrees for 20 to 30 minutes or until a meat thermometer registers 160 degrees for medium, basting occasionally with the pan juices.

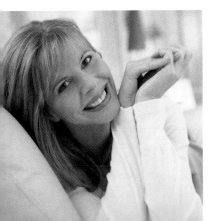

NUTRIENTS PER SERVING   Yield: 12 servings

CAL	PROT	CARBO	T FAT	SAT. FAT	MONOUFA	FIBER	SOD	OMEGA-3 FA	MG	K
163	23G	8G	4G	1G	2G	‹1G	78MG	‹1G	24MG	366MG

Pecan Pork Cutlets

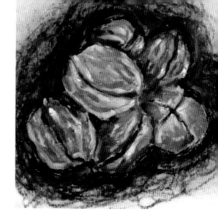

4	(4-ounce) pork loin cutlets
1/2	cup all-purpose flour
2	tablespoons unsalted butter or trans-fat-free margarine

1/4	cup honey
1/4	cup chopped pecans

Coat the cutlets with the flour, shaking off the excess. Heat 1 tablespoon of the butter in a heavy skillet over medium heat. Add the cutlets to the hot butter and cook for 5 to 6 minutes or until brown on both sides, turning occasionally.

Mix the remaining 1 tablespoon butter, honey and pecans in a bowl and add the butter mixture to the skillet, stirring gently. Simmer, covered, for 7 to 8 minutes or until the cutlets are cooked through. Remove the cutlets to a platter using a slotted spoon and drizzle with the sauce.

NUTRIENTS PER SERVING   Yield: 4 servings

CAL	PROT	CARBO	T FAT	SAT. FAT	MONOUFA	FIBER	SOD	OMEGA-3 FATS	MG	K
354	25G	30G	15G	5G	6G	1G	47MG	‹1G	35MG	409MG

Smothered Pork Chops

12	ounces fresh white mushrooms
1	tablespoon extra-virgin olive oil
2	large garlic cloves, cut into halves
4	(4-ounce) pork loin chops, 3/4 inch thick
1/2	cup dry white wine
1/2	teaspoon salt
1/4	teaspoon red pepper flakes (optional)
1	cup coarsely chopped plum tomatoes
1	tablespoon extra-virgin olive oil
1	large yellow or green bell pepper, cut into 1/4-inch strips
1	to 2 teaspoons water

Trim the mushroom stems and cut the mushrooms into thick slices. Heat 1 tablespoon olive oil in a skillet over medium heat until hot and add the garlic. Cook for 1 to 2 minutes or until golden brown; discard the garlic. Add the pork chops to the hot garlic oil and cook for 6 to 8 minutes or until light brown, turning once. Remove the pork chops to a platter using a slotted spoon and reserving the pan drippings.

Increase the heat to medium-high and add the wine, salt and red pepper flakes to the reserved pan drippings. Cook for 2 to 3 minutes or until the wine is reduced by 1/2, stirring with a wooden spoon to loosen any browned bits. Stir in the tomatoes and return the pork chops to the skillet. Reduce the heat to low and simmer, covered, for 15 minutes or until the chops register 160 degrees on a meat thermometer for medium.

Heat 1 tablespoon olive oil in a medium skillet over medium heat until hot. Add the mushrooms and bell pepper and cook for 5 minutes or until tender, stirring frequently. Add the mushroom mixture to the pork chops and mix well. Simmer, covered, for 3 minutes or just until hot, adding the water as needed for the desired consistency.

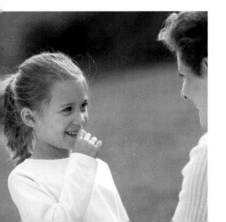

NUTRIENTS PER SERVING — Yield: 4 servings

CAL	PROT	CARBO	T FAT	SAT. FAT	MONOUFA	FIBER	SOD	OMEGA-3 FA	MG	K
282	27G	8G	14G	3G	8G	2G	346MG	<1G	28MG	787MG

Wild Rice-Stuffed Pork

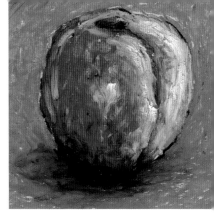

Wild Rice Stuffing

1	teaspoon butter or trans-fat-free margarine
1/3	cup chopped celery
1	tablespoon finely chopped green onion
1	cup cooked wild rice
1	tablespoon sliced almonds
1/4	teaspoon pepper
1/8	teaspoon salt

Pork

1/3	cup apricot preserves
1	tablespoon dry white wine
1/8	teaspoon ground cinnamon
4	(4-ounce) slices pork loin, 1 inch thick

For the stuffing, heat the butter in a skillet over medium heat and add the celery and green onion. Cook until the celery is tender-crisp, stirring frequently. Stir in the wild rice, almonds, pepper and salt.

For the pork, combine the preserves, wine and cinnamon in a bowl and mix well. Make a slit in the side of each loin slice cutting to but not through to form a pocket. Spoon about 1/3 cup of the stuffing into each pocket and secure with wooden picks.

Arrange the stuffed loin slices in an ungreased 8x8-inch baking dish and brush with the preserves mixture. Bake at 350 degrees for 40 to 45 minutes or until a meat thermometer registers 160 degrees for medium, brushing occasionally with the preserves mixture. Discard the wooden picks before serving.

Buckwheat is actually a fruit of a plant and is gluten-free. The roasted kernels make a good substitute for rice or pasta.

NUTRIENTS PER SERVING
Yield: 4 servings

CAL	PROT	CARBO	T FAT	SAT. FAT	MONOUFA	FIBER	SOD	OMEGA-3 FATS	MG	K
293	25G	27G	10G	3G	4G	1G	146MG	<1G	43MG	443MG

Dilled Chicken

Increase the lean protein serving slightly when omitting the bread serving at a meal.

2	tablespoons butter or trans-fat-free margarine
4	(4-ounce) boneless skinless chicken breasts
2	garlic cloves, minced
1	cup basmati rice

2	cups low-sodium chicken broth
1	tablespoon lemon juice
1	teaspoon grated lemon zest
2	tablespoons chopped fresh dill weed

Heat the butter in a 12-inch skillet over medium-high heat. Add the chicken to the butter and cook for 5 minutes or until brown on both sides, turning once. Remove the chicken to a platter using a slotted spoon, reserving the pan drippings.

Cook the garlic in the reserved pan drippings for 30 seconds, stirring constantly. Stir in the rice, broth, lemon juice and lemon zest. Bring to a boil and reduce the heat. Return the chicken to the skillet.

Simmer, covered, for 15 to 20 minutes or until the rice is tender, the liquid has been absorbed and the chicken is cooked through; do not stir. Stir in the dill weed and serve immediately.

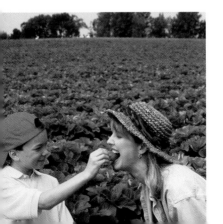

NUTRIENTS PER SERVING — Yield: 4 servings

CAL	PROT	CARBO	T FAT	SAT. FAT	MONOUFA	FIBER	SOD	OMEGA-3 FATS	MG	K
278	27G	21G	9G	5G	3G	1G	134MG	<1G	30MG	355MG

Cranberry Chicken

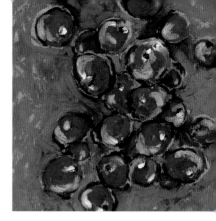

10 ounces fresh brussels sprouts, trimmed

1 tablespoon extra-virgin olive oil

1/4 teaspoon salt

1/4 teaspoon pepper

1 teaspoon extra-virgin olive oil

2 tablespoons all-purpose flour

1/4 teaspoon salt

1/4 teaspoon pepper

4 (4-ounce) boneless skinless chicken breasts

2 cups fresh cranberries

3/4 cup water

1/4 cup sugar

1/4 cup balsamic vinegar

Thinly slice the brussels sprouts and place on a 10×15-inch baking sheet with sides. Drizzle with 1 tablespoon olive oil and sprinkle with 1/4 teaspoon salt and 1/4 teaspoon pepper. Toss to coat and spread the sliced brussels sprouts in a single layer. Roast at 450 degrees for 15 to 20 minutes or until tender.

Heat 1 teaspoon olive oil in a 12-inch skillet over medium-high heat until hot. Mix the flour, 1/4 teaspoon salt and 1/4 teaspoon pepper on a sheet of waxed paper and coat the chicken with the flour mixture. Add the chicken to the hot oil and cook for 6 minutes; turn. Reduce the heat to medium and cook for 6 to 8 minutes longer or until the chicken is cooked through.

Remove the chicken to a platter using a slotted spoon, reserving the pan drippings. Cover to keep warm. Add the cranberries, water, sugar and vinegar to the reserved pan drippings and bring to a boil over medium-high heat, stirring occasionally. Cook for 5 minutes or until slightly thickened, stirring frequently. Serve the cranberry sauce with the chicken and roasted brussels sprouts.

NUTRIENTS PER SERVING   Yield: 4 servings

CAL	PROT	CARBO	T FAT	SAT. FAT	MONOUFA	FIBER	SOD	OMEGA-3 FA	MG	K
300	26G	33G	8G	1G	5G	5G	367MG	‹1G	41MG	520MG

Mushroom
Chicken Breasts

4   **(4-ounce) boneless skinless chicken breasts**

1   **teaspoon Italian seasoning**

1/2   **teaspoon garlic pepper**

1/2   **teaspoon paprika**

1/4   **cup white wine**

8   **ounces fresh mushrooms, sliced**

Sprinkle both sides of the chicken with the Italian seasoning, garlic pepper and paprika. Spray a large nonstick skillet with nonstick cooking spray and heat over medium heat until hot. Add the chicken to the hot skillet and cook for 3 minutes and turn.

Reduce the heat to medium-low and stir in the wine and mushrooms. Cook, covered, for 7 minutes longer or until a meat thermometer inserted in the chicken registers 170 degrees.

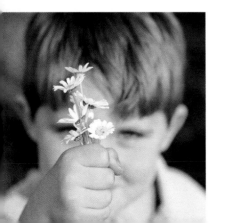

NUTRIENTS PER SERVING   Yield: 4 servings

CAL	PROT	CARBO	T FAT	SAT. FAT	MONOUFA	FIBER	SOD	OMEGA-3 FA	MG	K
146	25G	2G	3G	1G	1G	1G	58MG	<1G	29MG	410MG

Stuffed Chicken Breasts

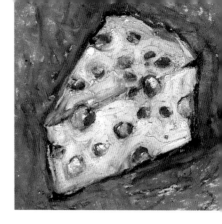

4 **(4-ounce) boneless skinless chicken breasts**	**¹/₄ cup chopped dry-roasted peanuts**
³/₄ cup (3 ounces) shredded part-skim mozzarella cheese	**Pepper to taste**
¹/₂ cup crumbled feta cheese	**Paprika to taste**

Using a sharp knife, make a pocket in each chicken breast by cutting from side to side, leaving the edges intact. Combine the mozzarella cheese, feta cheese and peanuts in a bowl and mix well.

Spoon the cheese mixture evenly into the pockets, packing lightly. Arrange the chicken in a single layer in a baking dish and sprinkle lightly with pepper and paprika. Bake at 350 degree for 50 to 55 minutes or until a meat thermometer registers 170 degrees.

Cut the fat in sandwiches and casseroles by using cheese made with 2% milk or other reduced-fat cheeses.

NUTRIENTS PER SERVING   Yield: 4 servings

CAL	PROT	CARBO	T FAT	SAT. FAT	MONOUFA	FIBER	SOD	OMEGA-3 FATS	MG	K
274	33G	3G	14G	6G	5G	1G	363MG	‹1G	44MG	273MG

Swiss Dijon Chicken Rolls

4   (4-ounce) boneless skinless chicken breasts

3/4 cup evaporated skim milk

2   tablespoons Dijon mustard

3/4 cup whole grain bread crumbs

1/2 cup (2 ounces) shredded Parmesan cheese

1 1/2 teaspoons tarragon

Pepper to taste

8   ounces reduced-fat Swiss cheese, shredded

Pound the chicken with a meat mallet between sheets of waxed paper until flattened. Mix the evaporated skim milk and Dijon mustard in a shallow dish until blended. Combine the bread crumbs, Parmesan cheese, tarragon and pepper in a shallow dish and mix well.

Sprinkle equal amounts of the Swiss cheese on each chicken breast and roll, beginning with the small end, to enclose the cheese. Dip each roll in the milk mixture and coat with the bread crumb mixture.

Arrange the rolls in a single layer in a baking pan sprayed with nonstick cooking spray. You may prepare to this point up to 1 day in advance and store, covered, in the refrigerator.

Bake, covered, in a convection oven at 375 degrees for 30 minutes. Remove the cover and bake for 15 minutes longer or until a meat thermometer registers 170 degrees.

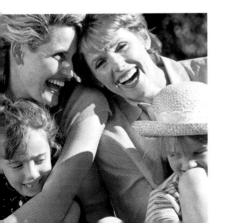

NUTRIENTS PER SERVING   Yield: 4 servings

CAL	PROT	CARBO	T FAT	SAT. FAT	MONOUFA	FIBER	SOD	OMEGA-3 FA	MG	K
332	47G	12G	10G	5G	3G	1G	643MG	<1G	65MG	443MG

Sun-Dried Tomato and Chicken Pasta

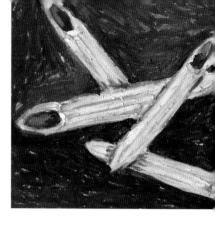

3/4 **cup boiling water**

1/4 **cup sun-dried tomato halves (not oil-pack)**

10 **ounces whole wheat bow tie pasta**

2 **teaspoons extra-virgin olive oil**

1 **red onion, chopped**

3 **garlic cloves, minced**

4 **(6-ounce) boneless skinless chicken breasts, cut into strips**

6 **ounces fresh mushrooms, sliced**

1/2 **cup dry white wine**

2 **tablespoons Dijon mustard**

3/4 **teaspoon oregano**

3 **tablespoons low-fat sour cream**

2 **tablespoons chopped fresh parsley**

Combine the boiling water and sun-dried tomatoes in a heatproof bowl and let stand for 20 minutes. Drain, reserving the liquid. Thinly slice the sun-dried tomatoes. Cook the pasta using package directions and drain. Cover to keep warm.

Heat the olive oil in a large nonstick skillet over medium heat. Add the onion and garlic and cook for 7 minutes or until the onion is tender. Stir in the chicken and mushrooms and cook for 4 minutes or until the chicken is golden brown, stirring constantly. Add the wine and increase the heat to high.

Cook for 2 minutes or until the chicken is cooked through and most of the liquid has evaporated, stirring constantly. Stir in the sun-dried tomatoes, reserved liquid, Dijon mustard and oregano and bring to a boil. Remove from the heat and stir in the sour cream and parsley. Toss the chicken mixture with the pasta in a bowl and serve immediately.

When cooking with wine, leave the pan uncovered so the alcohol will burn off. The resulting liquid will have a rounder, firmer, and fruitier flavor.

NUTRIENTS PER SERVING · Yield: 4 servings

CAL	PROT	CARBO	T FAT	SAT. FAT	MONOUFA	FIBER	SOD	OMEGA-3 FATS	MG	K
551	50G	63G	9G	2G	3G	2G	517MG	<1G	39MG	558MG

Cashew Chicken

1/2 **cup orange juice**	2 **tablespoons canola oil**
1/3 **cup honey**	4 **green onions, chopped**
1/4 **cup low-sodium soy sauce**	3 **large carrots, sliced**
1 **tablespoon cornstarch**	2 **ribs celery, sliced**
2 **garlic cloves, minced**	1 **pound boneless skinless chicken breasts, cut into 1-inch strips**
1 **teaspoon ground ginger**	
1/2 **teaspoon pepper**	1 **cup cashews**

Mix the orange juice, honey and soy sauce in a bowl and whisk in the cornstarch until blended. Add the garlic, ginger and pepper and mix well.

Heat 1 tablespoon of the canola oil in a skillet to the smoking point. Add the green onions, carrots and celery to the hot oil and stir-fry for several minutes or until the green onions are fragrant. Remove the vegetable mixture to a platter.

Heat the remaining 1 tablespoon canola oil in the skillet to the smoking point and add the chicken. Stir-fry until the chicken is brown and cooked through. Return the vegetable mixture to the skillet and mix well. Stir in the orange juice mixture and cashews and cook until thickened, stirring constantly. Spoon over hot cooked brown rice on serving plates.

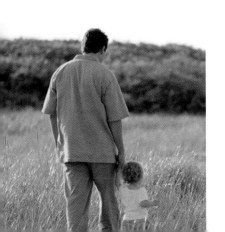

NUTRIENTS PER SERVING   Yield: 4 servings

CAL	PROT	CARBO	T FAT	SAT. FAT	MONOUFA	FIBER	SOD	OMEGA-3 FA	MG	K
521	31G	46G	25G	4G	13G	3G	721MG	1G	126MG	743MG

Nutritional profile does not include brown rice.

Sweet Onion Barbecued
Chicken Sandwiches

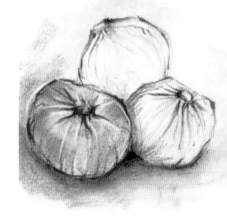

1	**tablespoon extra-virgin olive oil**
2	**cups finely chopped sweet onions**
3	**tablespoon cider vinegar**
1	**tablespoon brown sugar**
3	**cups chopped cooked boneless skinless chicken breasts**

1/2	**cup barbecue sauce**
2	**tablespoons water**
1/4	**teaspoon pepper**
6	**multigrain buns, split**
1	**tablespoon extra-virgin olive oil**

Heat 1 tablespoon olive oil in a 10-inch skillet over medium-low heat and add the onions. Cook for 7 minutes and stir in the vinegar and brown sugar. Cook for 2 minutes and stir in the chicken, barbecue sauce, water and pepper. Cook for 5 minutes longer or until heated through, stirring occasionally.

Arrange the buns cut side up on a baking sheet and brush the cut sides with 1 tablespoon olive oil. Broil until golden brown. Spoon the barbecued chicken over the cut side of each bun. Serve open-faced.

When grilling sandwiches such as grilled cheese, spray the bread slices with canola nonstick cooking spray or olive oil nonstick cooking spray instead of brushing them with butter.

NUTRIENTS PER SERVING — Yield: 6 servings

CAL	PROT	CARBO	T FAT	SAT. FAT	MONOUFA	FIBER	SOD	OMEGA-3 FATS	MG	K
355	29G	35G	11G	2G	6G	4G	454MG	‹1G	32MG	308MG

Stuffed Turkey Breast

1	**(3-pound) turkey breast, boned with skin intact**
2	**tablespoons chopped fresh thyme, or 1¹/₂ teaspoons dried thyme**
¹/₂	**teaspoon salt**
¹/₂	**teaspoon freshly ground pepper**
¹/₂	**teaspoon ground cinnamon**
¹/₂	**teaspoon ground allspice**
¹/₂	**teaspoon cardamom**
4	**cups Corn Bread Stuffing (page 78)**
¹/₂	**cup apple cider**
2	**tablespoons butter or trans-fat-free margarine, melted**

Place the turkey skin side down on a hard work surface. Cover with waxed paper and pound with a meat mallet if not uniform in thickness. Combine the thyme, salt, pepper, cinnamon, allspice and cardamom in a bowl and mix well. Rub the thyme mixture over the skinless side. Roll the turkey breast skin side out. Wrap in plastic wrap and chill for 4 to 10 hours.

Unroll the turkey breast and spoon the stuffing down the center. Bring both sides of the turkey breast together to enclose the stuffing, tucking 1 side under the other to form a tight roll approximately 5 inches in diameter. Secure with kitchen twine or skewers. Arrange the turkey roll seam side down in a roasting pan and cover with foil.

Roast at 400 degrees for 40 minutes and reduce the oven temperature to 350 degrees. Remove the foil and roast for 20 minutes longer or until a meat thermometer registers 170 degrees and the juices run clear when lightly pricked with a fork, basting with a mixture of the apple cider and butter several times.

Remove the turkey from the oven and let stand for 15 minutes. Remove the twine and skin and cut into ¹/₄- to ¹/₂-inch slices. Serve with the pan juices and additional baked stuffing if desired.

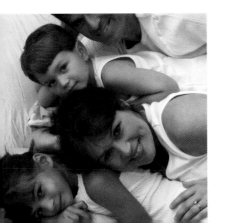

NUTRIENTS PER SERVING — Yield: 12 servings

CAL	PROT	CARBO	T FAT	SAT. FAT	MONOUFA	FIBER	SOD	OMEGA-3 FA	MG	K
291	30G	25G	7G	3G	2G	4G	527MG	‹1G	41MG	377MG

Blackened Fish

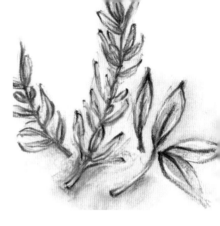

1	tablespoon paprika	1/2	teaspoon thyme
1	teaspoon salt	1/2	teaspoon oregano
1	teaspoon onion powder	1/8	teaspoon ground cumin
1	teaspoon garlic powder	2	pounds sole fillets, 1/2 to 3/4 inch thick
3/4	teaspoon cayenne pepper		
1/2	teaspoon black pepper	1/3	cup extra-virgin olive oil
1/2	teaspoon white pepper		

Mix the paprika, salt, onion powder, garlic powder, cayenne pepper, black pepper, white pepper, thyme, oregano and cumin in a bowl. Brush the fillets with the olive oil and coat with the paprika mixture, patting lightly to make sure the herb mixture adheres.

Arrange the fillets in a single layer in a skillet sprayed with nonstick cooking spray. Cook over medium-high heat for 2 to 3 minutes per side or until charred or blackened, turning once. The blackening forms a spicy, crunchy coating that seals in the moisture and flavor.

Make healthier "refried" beans by mashing black or pinto beans with your favorite spices such as ground cumin and cayenne pepper.

NUTRIENTS PER SERVING Yield: 6 servings

CAL	PROT	CARBO	T FAT	SAT. FAT	MONOUFA	FIBER	SOD	OMEGA-3 FATS	MG	K
237	25G	1G	14G	2G	10G	‹1G	497MG	1G	62MG	384MG

Just two servings of fish per week reduce the risk of dying from a heart attack by thirty to fifty percent.

Salmon Fillets with Fresh Mango Salsa

4	**(6-ounce) salmon fillets, 1 inch thick**	**1/2**	**teaspoon salt**
1/4	**cup chopped fresh cilantro**	**1/4**	**teaspoon black pepper**
1/4	**cup chopped fresh mint**	**1/8**	**teaspoon ground red pepper**
1	**teaspoon extra-virgin olive oil**	**11/3**	**cups Fresh Mango Salsa (page 103)**

Place the fillets in a sealable plastic bag. Add the cilantro, mint and olive oil to the bag and seal tightly. Shake gently to coat. Marinate in the refrigerator for 20 minutes, turning once or twice.

Remove the fillets from the bag and sprinkle with the salt, black pepper and red pepper. Arrange the fillets on a grill rack coated with nonstick cooking spray and grill for 5 minutes per side or until the fillets flake easily. Serve with the Fresh Mango Salsa and hot cooked brown rice.

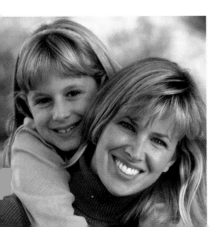

NUTRIENTS PER SERVING — Yield: 4 servings

CAL	PROT	CARBO	T FAT	SAT. FAT	MONOUFA	FIBER	SOD	OMEGA-3 FA	MG	K
358	39G	11G	17G	3G	8G	1G	385MG	2G	57MG	686MG

Nutritional profile does not include brown rice.

Fresh Mango Salsa

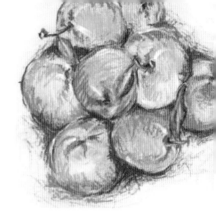

1   (8-ounce) can juice-pack pineapple chunks, drained

1   cup chopped peeled mango

1   cup chopped banana

1/4 cup chopped fresh mint

2   tablespoons fresh orange juice

1   tablespoon fresh lime juice

1   serrano chile, seeded and finely chopped

Combine the pineapple, mango, banana, mint, orange juice, lime juice and serrano chile in a bowl and mix well. Chill, covered, in the refrigerator until serving time. Serve as an accompaniment with fish, pork or chicken or as a dip with baked chips.

NUTRIENTS PER 1/3 CUP   Yield: 8 (1/3-cup) servings

CAL	PROT	CARBO	T FAT	SAT. FAT	MONOUFA	FIBER	SOD	OMEGA-3 FATS	MG	K
42	1G	11G	<1G	<1G	<1G	1G	1MG	<1G	13MG	148MG

Glazed Salmon

Honey Mustard Glaze

2	tablespoons honey
2	tablespoons warm water
2	teaspoons soy sauce
1/8	teaspoon dry mustard
	Salt and pepper to taste

Salmon

4	(6-ounce) salmon fillets
1	tablespoon extra-virgin olive oil
1/16	teaspoon salt
1/16	teaspoon pepper

For the glaze, combine the honey, warm water, soy sauce, dry mustard, salt and pepper in a bowl and mix well.

For the salmon, brush both sides of the fillets with the olive oil and sprinkle with the salt and pepper. Arrange the fillets on a grill rack and grill for 2 to 3 minutes or until grill marks appear and turn. Grill until the fillets flake easily; do not turn. Brush the fillets with the glaze just before removing from the grill and serve immediately.

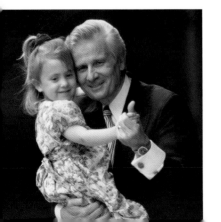

NUTRIENTS PER SERVING   Yield: 4 servings

CAL	PROT	CARBO	T FAT	SAT. FAT	MONOUFA	FIBER	SOD	OMEGA-3 FA	MG	K
371	39G	9G	19G	3G	10G	‹1G	349MG	2G	44MG	536MG

Salmon Loaf

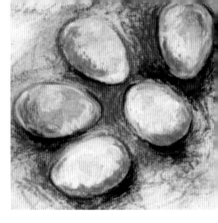

2	**cups canned salmon**	**1/3**	**cup chopped onion**
1	**cup soft whole wheat bread crumbs**	**2**	**teaspoons lemon juice**
3	**Omega-3-enhanced eggs, beaten**	**1**	**teaspoon chopped fresh parsley**
2	**tablespoons butter or trans-fat-free margarine, melted**		**Sprigs of parsley**
			Lemon wedges

Drain the salmon, reserving 1/4 cup of the liquid. Flake the salmon in a bowl. Add the reserved liquid, bread crumbs, eggs, butter, onion, lemon juice and chopped parsley to the salmon and mix well.

Shape the salmon mixture into a loaf in a greased 5x9-inch loaf pan. Bake, covered, at 300 degrees for 1 hour. Garnish with sprigs of parsley and lemon wedges.

Fatty fish like salmon and tuna are excellent sources of essential Omega-3 fatty acids.

NUTRIENTS PER SERVING — Yield: 6 servings

CAL	PROT	CARBO	T FAT	SAT. FAT	MONOUFA	FIBER	SOD	OMEGA-3 FATS	MG	K
163	14G	5G	9G	3G	3G	1G	383MG	1G	28MG	235MG

Grilled Tuna with
Cherry Tomato Salsa

4	(6-ounce) tuna, salmon or halibut steaks with bone		2	cups cherry or pear tomatoes, cut into halves
1	tablespoon extra-virgin olive oil		1/2	teaspoon salt
1	tablespoon lemon juice		2	tablespoons chopped fresh flat-leaf parsley
1/4	cup finely chopped red onion		1	tablespoon drained capers (optional)
2	garlic cloves, minced			Freshly ground pepper to taste
2	teaspoons extra-virgin olive oil			

Rinse the steaks and pat dry with paper towels. Arrange the steaks in a single layer in a round glass dish and drizzle with 1 tablespoon olive oil and the lemon juice, turning to coat. Marinate, covered, in the refrigerator for 15 minutes to 4 hours.

Spray a heavy-duty sheet of foil with nonstick cooking spray and arrange the steaks on the prepared foil. Place on the grill rack and grill over hot coals for 4 to 8 minutes per side or until the steaks flake easily and the center is not quite opaque, turning once. Remove the steaks to a platter and cover to keep warm.

Combine the onion, garlic and 2 teaspoons olive oil in a round baking dish and roast at 400 degrees for 7 to 8 minutes, stirring halfway through the roasting process. Toss the tomatoes and salt in a bowl and add to the onion mixture. Roast for 4 to 5 minutes longer or until the tomatoes are heated through and the onion begins to brown. Remove from the oven and stir in the parsley and capers. Spoon the onion mixture over the tuna steaks and sprinkle with pepper. Serve immediately.

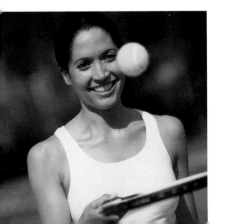

NUTRIENTS PER SERVING   Yield: 4 servings

CAL	PROT	CARBO	T FAT	SAT. FAT	MONOUFA	FIBER	SOD	OMEGA-3 FA	MG	K
327	42G	5G	15G	3G	7G	1G	367MG	2G	98MG	641MG

Corn Bread
Black Bean Casserole

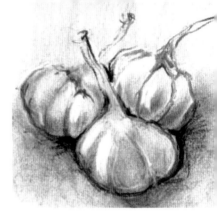

Black Bean Casserole

1	cup chopped onion
1	large garlic clove, minced
1	tablespoon extra-virgin olive oil
1	large green bell pepper, chopped
1	large rib celery, finely chopped
1	carrot, finely chopped
1	(15-ounce) can black beans, drained and rinsed
1	(14-ounce) can diced tomatoes with green chiles, drained
1/2	teaspoon oregano
1/2	cup packed minced fresh cilantro

Corn Bread Topping and Assembly

1	cup yellow cornmeal
1/3	cup unbleached all-purpose flour
1/2	teaspoon baking powder
1/4	teaspoon baking soda
1/4	teaspoon salt
1/2	cup fresh or frozen corn
1	cup buttermilk
1	tablespoon canola oil
1	tablespoon maple syrup

Substitute cream-style corn for the oil in corn bread recipes.

For the casserole, sauté the onion and garlic in the olive oil in a nonstick skillet over medium heat for 2 minutes. Stir in the bell pepper, celery and carrot and sauté for 5 minutes. Mix in the next 3 ingredients. Cook for 5 minutes or until the vegetables begin to soften. Remove from the heat and stir in the cilantro. Spoon the bean mixture into a shallow round 3-quart baking dish sprayed with nonstick cooking spray.

For the topping, mix the cornmeal, flour, baking powder, baking soda and salt in a bowl and stir in the corn. Blend the buttermilk, canola oil and syrup in a bowl and add to the cornmeal mixture, stirring just until moistened. Spread the topping over the prepared layer and bake at 400 degrees for 30 to 35 minutes or until a wooden pick inserted in the center comes out clean. Cut into wedges.

NUTRIENTS PER SERVING   Yield: 6 servings

CAL	PROT	CARBO	T FAT	SAT. FAT	MONOUFA	FIBER	SOD	OMEGA-3 FATS	MG	K
265	9G	47G	6G	1G	4G	8G	786MG	<1G	53MG	400MG

Layered Enchilada Bake

1½ cups brown rice

8 ounces hot pepper cheese, shredded

1 cup low-fat cottage cheese

½ cup fat-free sour cream

½ cup chopped onion

2 teaspoons chili powder

2 teaspoons ground cumin

6 (10-inch) whole wheat tortillas

2 cups rinsed and drained canned black beans

½ cup chopped tomato

1 teaspoon minced fresh cilantro

1½ cups (6 ounces) shredded part-skim mozzarella cheese

1⅓ cups salsa

Cook the brown rice using package directions. Combine the brown rice, hot pepper cheese, cottage cheese, sour cream, onion, chili powder and cumin in a bowl and mix well.

Line the bottom of a 9×13-inch baking dish sprayed with nonstick cooking spray with 2 of the tortillas and spread with 3 cups of the brown rice mixture. Repeat the layering process 2 more times and top with the beans, spreading to the edges. Sprinkle with the tomato, cilantro and mozzarella cheese. Bake at 350 degrees for 30 to 45 minutes or until brown and bubbly. Garnish with the salsa.

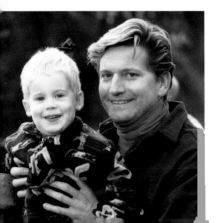

NUTRIENTS PER SERVING   Yield: 12 servings

CAL	PROT	CARBO	T FAT	SAT. FAT	MONOUFA	FIBER	SOD	OMEGA-3 FA	MG	K
305	17G	41G	10G	6G	1G	5G	661MG	<1G	57MG	264MG

Red Lentil Burritos

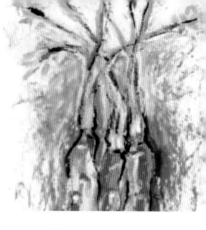

1 **cup boiling water**	1/2 **cup cauliflower florets, chopped**
8 **dry-pack sun-dried tomatoes**	1/2 **cup thinly sliced carrots**
2 1/2 **cups water**	1/2 **cup canned tomato sauce**
1 **cup red lentils, sorted and rinsed**	1 **teaspoon curry powder**
1 **tablespoon extra-virgin olive oil**	1/2 **teaspoon ground cinnamon**
1/2 **cup chopped onion**	4 **(8-inch) whole wheat tortillas, heated**
1/2 **cup broccoli florets, chopped**	

Pour 1 cup boiling water over the sun-dried tomatoes in a heatproof bowl and let stand for 10 minutes or until soft. Drain, reserving 1/2 cup of the liquid. Chop the sun-dried tomatoes.

Combine 2 1/2 cups water, the lentils and reserved liquid in a medium saucepan. Bring to a boil over medium-high heat and reduce the heat to low. Simmer for 6 to 10 minutes or just until the lentils are tender; drain.

Heat the olive oil in a nonstick skillet over medium heat. Add the onion, broccoli, cauliflower and carrots to the hot oil and sauté for 4 to 5 minutes or until the vegetables are tender. Stir in the tomato sauce, curry powder and cinnamon. Add the lentils and sun-dried tomatoes and simmer for 15 to 20 minutes or until slightly thickened, stirring occasionally. Spoon equal portions of the lentil mixture on the warm tortillas and roll to enclose the filling.

Cook dried beans slowly to retain their shape and texture and to avoid their burning and sticking to the bottom of the stockpot. The darker the dried bean, the stronger the flavor.

NUTRIENTS PER BURRITO

Yield: 4 burritos

CAL	PROT	CARBO	T FAT	SAT. FAT	MONOUFA	FIBER	SOD	OMEGA-3 FATS	MG	K
327	17G	63G	5G	1G	3G	13G	707MG	‹1G	70MG	1249MG

Pesto Fettuccini

Substitute white wine or water for chicken broth for a healthier alternative.

Basil Pesto

1   **cup packed fresh basil leaves**

3   **tablespoons grated Parmesan cheese**

2   **tablespoons extra-virgin olive oil**

2   **tablespoons soy nuts**

3   **garlic cloves, minced**

Fettuccini and Assembly

12   **ounces fettuccini**

2   **cups frozen broccoli and cauliflower**

1   **cup low-sodium chicken broth**

1   **tablespoon lite cream cheese**

For the pesto, combine the basil, cheese, olive oil, soy nuts and garlic in a food processor or blender and process until puréed.

For the fettuccini, cook the pasta using package directions, adding the broccoli and cauliflower 3 minutes before the end of the cooking process; drain. Cover to keep warm.

Bring the broth to a simmer in a large nonstick skillet over medium heat. Whisk in the pesto and cream cheese until smooth. Add the pasta mixture and cook for 2 minutes or until heated through, stirring frequently. Serve with roasted chicken breasts.

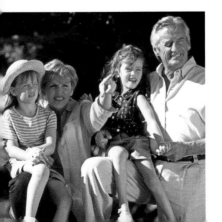

NUTRIENTS PER SERVING   Yield: 6 servings

CAL	PROT	CARBO	T FAT	SAT. FAT	MONOUFA	FIBER	SOD	OMEGA-3 FA	MG	K
360	17G	57G	8G	2G	4G	10G	85MG	‹1G	32MG	129MG

Greek **Lasagna**

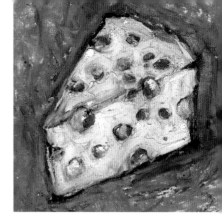

3	(10-ounce) packages spinach, thawed and drained	2	tablespoons all-purpose flour
1	tablespoon extra-virgin olive oil	8	ounces feta cheese, crumbled
2	onions, chopped	2	Omega-3-enhanced egg whites, slightly beaten
3	garlic cloves, minced	1	pound phyllo pastry
2	tablespoons chopped fresh dill weed	2	tablespoons unsalted butter or trans-fat-free margarine, melted

Press the excess moisture from the spinach. Heat the olive oil in a large skillet and add the onions and garlic. Cook until the onions are tender, stirring frequently. Stir in the spinach, dill weed and flour and cook for 10 minutes or until most of the moisture has evaporated, stirring frequently. Remove from the heat and stir in the cheese and egg whites.

Layer 1/3 of the phyllo in a 9×13-inch baking pan sprayed with nonstick cooking spray and brush with 1/3 of the butter. Spread with 1/3 of the spinach mixture. Repeat the process 2 more times with the remaining phyllo, remaining butter and remaining spinach mixture. Bake at 350 degrees for 30 minutes.

NUTRIENTS PER SERVING   Yield: 12 servings

CAL	PROT	CARBO	T FAT	SAT. FAT	MONOUFA	FIBER	SOD	OMEGA-3 FATS	MG	K
229	9G	27G	10G	5G	3G	3G	456MG	<1G	64MG	344MG

Stuffed **Bell Peppers**

1²/₃ cups reduced-sodium vegetable broth	¹/₂ cup shredded carrots
³/₄ cup brown rice	2 garlic cloves, minced
¹/₄ cup wild rice	1 teaspoon ground cumin
4 red, yellow or green bell peppers	¹/₂ cup (2 ounces) shredded reduced-fat mozzarella cheese
¹/₄ cup chopped onion	1¹/₂ teaspoons chopped fresh basil
1 tablespoon extra-virgin olive oil	4 thin slices reduced-fat mozzarella cheese
¹/₂ cup fresh or frozen peas	
¹/₂ cup fresh or frozen corn	1 cup canned tomato sauce, heated

Mix the broth, brown rice and wild rice in a saucepan and bring to a boil over medium heat. Reduce the heat and simmer, covered, for 20 minutes or until the rice is tender and the broth has been absorbed. Cut 1 inch off the top of each bell pepper and discard the tops. Remove the seeds and membranes carefully. Trim the bottoms if necessary to allow the bell peppers to stand upright. Blanch the bell peppers in gently boiling water in a saucepan for 6 minutes or until tender but still retain their shape; drain.

Sauté the onion in the olive oil in a skillet for 4 minutes or until tender. Stir in the peas, corn, carrots, garlic and cumin. Reduce the heat to low and simmer, covered, for 5 minutes. Remove from the heat and stir in the rice mixture, shredded mozzarella cheese and basil. Stuff the bell peppers with the rice mixture and top each with 1 slice of mozzarella cheese. Arrange the bell peppers in an 8×8-inch baking dish. Add enough water to the baking dish to measure ¹/₄ inch and bake at 375 degrees for 15 minutes or until heated through. Broil 6 inches from the heat source for 3 minutes or until the cheese is bubbly and light brown. Serve with the warm tomato sauce.

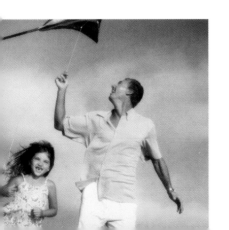

NUTRIENTS PER SERVING Yield: 4 servings

CAL	PROT	CARBO	T FAT	SAT. FAT	MONOUFA	FIBER	SOD	OMEGA-3 FA	MG	K
406	20G	57G	13G	5G	3G	6G	670MG	<1G	113MG	715MG

Vegetarian Jambalaya

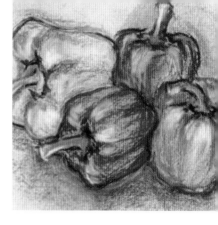

1	tablespoon canola oil	1	cup bulgur
1	cup chopped onion	3/4	teaspoon thyme
1/2	cup chopped celery	1/4	teaspoon ground red pepper
1/2	cup chopped green bell pepper	1/4	cup low-sodium vegetable broth
2	garlic cloves, minced	1	(19-ounce) can red kidney beans, drained and rinsed
1	cup salsa	1	cup drained canned corn
1	cup reduced-sodium tomato sauce	1/4	cup low-sodium vegetable broth

Heat the canola oil in a large nonstick skillet over medium heat. Add the onion, celery, bell pepper and garlic to the hot oil and sauté for 5 minutes or until the vegetables are tender. Stir in the salsa, tomato sauce, bulgur, thyme, red pepper and 1/4 cup broth.

Bring to a boil and reduce the heat to low. Simmer, covered, for 10 minutes. Stir in the beans, corn and 1/4 cup broth and simmer, covered, for 5 to 10 minutes longer or until the bulgur is tender.

Lower your cholesterol and stay full longer by increasing your fiber intake.

NUTRIENTS PER SERVING — Yield: 8 servings

CAL	PROT	CARBO	T FAT	SAT. FAT	MONOUFA	FIBER	SOD	OMEGA-3 FATS	MG	K
179	7G	34G	3G	‹1G	1G	8G	457MG	‹1G	66MG	549MG

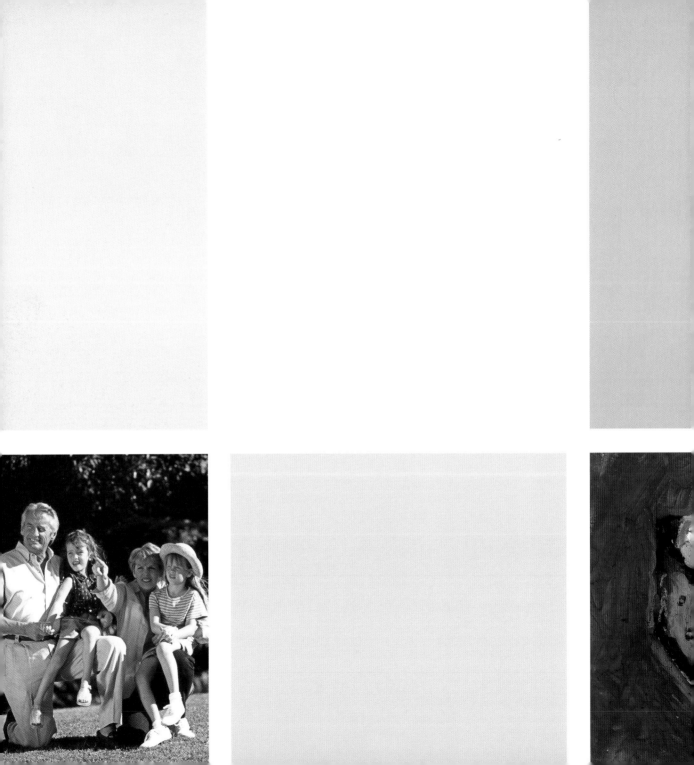

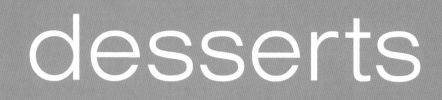

desserts

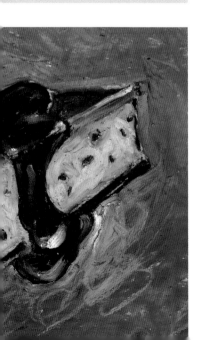

Everyone loves a happy ending. These desserts are sure to put a smile on your face at the end of a meal, or as an anytime treat. If you are craving chocolate or something fruity, you can find healthy recipes to satisfy your sweet tooth.

Tropical Breezer

1 or 2 ripe bananas, chopped

3 peaches, peeled and chopped

1 cup drained pineapple in lite syrup

1 cup unsweetened pineapple juice

3 tablespoons toasted wheat germ

2 tablespoons honey

6 or 7 ice cubes

Combine the bananas, peaches, pineapple, pineapple juice, wheat germ, honey and ice in a blender. Process on medium-high for 45 seconds or until smooth. Pour into glasses and serve immediately. You may substitute 1 drained 15-ounce can peaches in lite syrup for the fresh peaches.

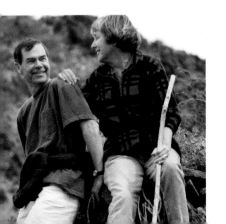

NUTRIENTS PER SERVING									Yield: 4 servings	
CAL	PROT	CARBO	T FAT	SAT. FAT	MONOUFA	FIBER	SOD	OMEGA-3 FA	MG	K
201	3G	49G	1G	‹1G	‹1G	4G	2MG	‹1G	58MG	556MG

Orange **Cream Smoothie**

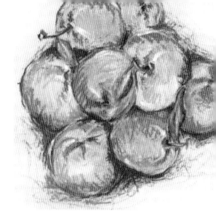

3   **cups fat-free vanilla ice cream or frozen yogurt**

1¹/₂ **cups fresh orange juice or orange juice with pulp**

¹/₄ **cup ground flaxseed**

3   **tablespoons honey**

Combine the ice cream, orange juice, flaxseed and honey in a blender. Process on medium-high for 45 seconds or until smooth. Pour into glasses and serve immediately.

Two medium kiwifruit have more potassium (505 milligrams) than a banana, and twice the vitamin C (114 milligrams) and fiber (5 milligrams) of a small orange.

NUTRIENTS PER SERVING   Yield: 6 servings

CAL	PROT	CARBO	T FAT	SAT. FAT	MONOUFA	FIBER	SOD	OMEGA-3 FATS	MG	K
187	5G	38G	2G	‹1G	‹1G	2G	53MG	1G	27MG	166MG

desserts

Melon and Berries with Almond Cream

1/2 cup fat-free cream cheese, softened	1/2 cantaloupe, sliced
2 tablespoons confectioners' sugar	1 cup fresh blackberries
1 tablespoon 1% milk	1 tablespoon sliced almonds, toasted
1/4 teaspoon almond extract	

Combine the cream cheese, confectioners' sugar, 1% milk and flavoring in a mixing bowl and beat at high speed until smooth. Arrange the cantaloupe, blackberries and cream cheese mixture on 4 dessert plates and sprinkle with the almonds.

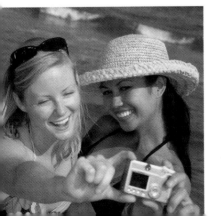

NUTRIENTS PER SERVING   Yield: 4 servings

CAL	PROT	CARBO	T FAT	SAT. FAT	MONOUFA	FIBER	SOD	OMEGA-3 FA	MG	K
95	7G	15G	1G	‹1G	1G	3G	174MG	‹1G	21MG	325MG

Chocolate Almond Cheesecake

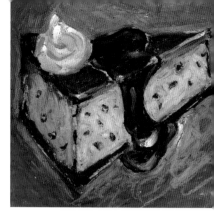

16	ounces fat-free cream cheese, softened		1	tablespoon unsweetened baking cocoa
16	ounces cream cheese, softened		2	teaspoons vanilla extract
1	cup artificial sweetener		1	teaspoon almond extract
1	cup sugar		1	cup (6 ounces) chocolate chips, melted
4	Omega-3-enhanced eggs		1/2	cup blanched chopped almonds

Combine the fat-free cream cheese, cream cheese, artificial sweetener and sugar in a mixing bowl and beat at medium speed for 3 to 4 minutes or until light and fluffy, scraping the bowl frequently. Add the eggs 1 at a time, beating constantly until creamy after each addition. This process should take 1 to 2 minutes.

Add the baking cocoa and flavorings to the cream cheese mixture and beat for 1 to 2 minutes longer or until blended. Fold in the melted chocolate chips until swirled throughout the mixture.

Sprinkle the almonds over the bottom of a lightly buttered 9-inch springform pan. Spread the cream cheese mixture in the prepared pan and bake at 325 degrees for 65 to 75 minutes or until set. Turn off the oven and let the cheesecake stand in the oven with the door closed for 2 hours. Remove the side of the pan and cool completely on a wire rack. Chill, covered, for 8 to 10 hours. Store leftovers in the refrigerator.

NUTRIENTS PER SERVING — Yield: 12 servings

CAL	PROT	CARBO	T FAT	SAT. FAT	MONOUFA	FIBER	SOD	OMEGA-3 FATS	MG	K
357	12G	33G	21G	12G	4G	2G	334MG	<1G	33MG	246MG

Autumn Crisp

Brown Sugar and Oat Topping

- **¹/₃ cup butter or trans-fat-free margarine, softened**
- **¹/₂ cup all-purpose flour**
- **¹/₄ cup whole wheat flour**
- **¹/₂ cup old-fashioned oats**
- **¹/₂ cup packed brown sugar**

Crisp

- **3 cups sliced peeled apples**
- **2 cups sliced peeled pears**
- **1 cup fresh cranberries**
- **3 tablespoons quick-cooking tapioca**
- **1 cup water**
- **1¹/₄ cups sugar**
- **¹/₂ teaspoon ground cinnamon**

For the topping, combine the butter, all-purpose flour, whole wheat flour, oats and brown sugar in a bowl and mix until crumbly.

For the crisp, combine the apples, pears, cranberries and tapioca in a large saucepan and mix well. Stir in the water and bring to a boil over medium heat. Cook until the cranberries begin to pop and stir in the sugar and cinnamon. Return the apple mixture to a boil and boil for 1 minute, stirring constantly.

Spoon the apple mixture into a 2-quart baking dish and sprinkle with the topping. Bake at 375 degrees for 30 minutes or until golden brown and bubbly.

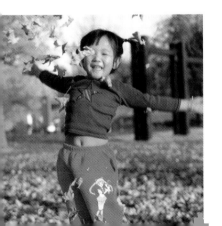

NUTRIENTS PER SERVING **Yield: 12 servings**

CAL	PROT	CARBO	T FAT	SAT. FAT	MONOUFA	FIBER	SOD	OMEGA-3 FA	MG	K
239	2G	48G	6G	3G	1G	2G	40MG	‹1G	16MG	129MG

Baked Pears

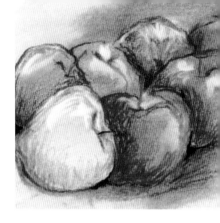

4	pears
2	tablespoons all-purpose flour
2	tablespoons brown sugar
1/16	teaspoon ground nutmeg

| 1 | tablespoon extra-virgin olive oil or canola oil |
| 1 | tablespoon sliced almonds |

Cut the pears lengthwise into halves and core. Arrange the pears cut side down in a 9×13-inch baking dish sprayed with nonstick cooking spray. Bake at 350 degrees for 25 minutes. Maintain the oven temperature.

Combine the flour, brown sugar and nutmeg in a small bowl and mix well. Add the olive oil and mix with a fork until crumbly. Stir in the almonds. Turn the pears cut side up and sprinkle with the almond mixture. Bake for 20 minutes longer or until the pears are tender and the crumb topping is brown.

Certified organic products are raised and processed without pesticides, herbicides, and fertilizers.

NUTRIENTS PER SERVING   Yield: 4 servings

CAL	PROT	CARBO	T FAT	SAT. FAT	MONOUFA	FIBER	SOD	OMEGA-3 FATS	MG	K
181	2G	35G	5G	1G	3G	4G	3MG	<1G	7MG	249MG

Cranberry Almond Dessert

Use a full-spectrum multivitamin to "fill in the cracks" of your healthy diet.

2/3	cup sugar	1	(12-ounce) package lite extra-firm silken tofu
2	tablespoons cornstarch	1/3	cup sugar
3	cups fresh cranberries	1/2	teaspoon vanilla extract
1/4	cup water	1/4	teaspoon almond extract
2	tablespoons unsweetened orange juice	13/4	cups almonds, chopped

Combine 2/3 cup sugar and the cornstarch in a saucepan and mix well. Stir in the cranberries, water and orange juice. Bring to a boil and boil for 1 minute, stirring constantly. Remove from the heat and let stand until cool.

Drain the tofu. Wrap the tofu in a paper towel and squeeze to remove any remaining moisture. Combine the tofu, 1/3 cup sugar and the flavorings in a blender and process until smooth. Pour equal portions of the tofu mixture into dessert bowls and drizzle with the cooled cranberry sauce. Chill, covered, until serving time. Sprinkle with the almonds just before serving.

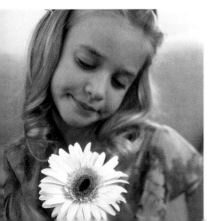

NUTRIENTS PER SERVING   Yield: 16 servings

CAL	PROT	CARBO	T FAT	SAT. FAT	MONOUFA	FIBER	SOD	OMEGA-3 FA	MG	K
161	5G	19G	8G	1G	5G	2G	26MG	<1G	47MG	140MG

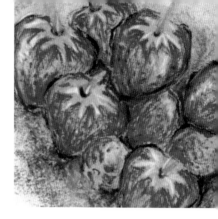

Raspberry
Chocolate Soufflé

1/4 **cup (1/2 stick) unsalted butter**	1 **Omega-3-enhanced egg yolk**
3 **ounces semisweet chocolate, chopped**	2 **tablespoons brown sugar**
	2 **teaspoons all-purpose flour**
1 **Omega-3-enhanced egg**	1 **cup fresh raspberries**

Combine the butter and chocolate in a small saucepan and cook just until the chocolate is almost melted, stirring frequently. Remove from the heat and stir until smooth. Let stand until room temperature.

Combine the egg, egg yolk and brown sugar in a mixing bowl and beat for 3 to 4 minutes or until the mixture is thick and pale yellow in color or until a ribbon-like pattern forms when the beaters are lifted. Add the chocolate mixture and beat until blended. Fold in the flour.

Spoon equal portions of the chocolate batter into 8 greased 6-ounce custard cups. Sprinkle evenly with the raspberries and arrange the custard cups on a baking sheet. Bake at 450 degrees for 12 minutes. Garnish with confectioners' sugar. Serve warm.

NUTRIENTS PER SERVING   Yield: 8 servings

CAL	PROT	CARBO	T FAT	SAT. FAT	MONOUFA	FIBER	SOD	OMEGA-3 FATS	MG	K
138	2G	12G	10G	6G	2G	2G	12MG	<1G	6MG	101MG

Chocolate
Microwave Pudding

6	**tablespoons sugar**	**1 1/2 cups skim milk**	
1/4	**cup unsweetened baking cocoa**	**1/2 teaspoon vanilla extract**	
2	**tablespoons cornstarch**		

Combine the sugar, baking cocoa and cornstarch in a 1-quart microwave-safe bowl and mix well. Add the skim milk gradually, whisking constantly until blended.

Microwave on High for 3 minutes, stirring halfway through the process. Microwave on Medium-High (70%) for 1 1/2 minutes longer or until thickened. Whisk in the vanilla. Serve warm or chilled in dessert bowls.

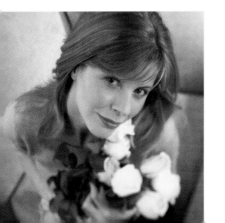

NUTRIENTS PER 1/2 CUP — Yield: 3 (1/2-cup) servings

CAL	PROT	CARBO	T FAT	SAT. FAT	MONOUFA	FIBER	SOD	OMEGA-3 FA	MG	K
179	5G	40G	1G	<1G	1G	1G	52MG	<1G	14MG	309MG

Rice **Pudding**

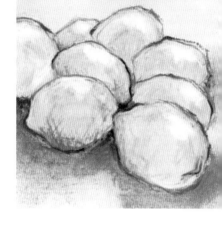

1 tablespoon butter or trans-fat-free margarine, softened	2 cups cooked brown or long grain rice
1/2 cup packed brown sugar	1 teaspoon fresh lemon juice
1 1/3 cups skim milk	1/2 teaspoon grated lemon zest
4 Omega-3-enhanced eggs	1/3 cup chopped dried fruit (dates, raisins or dried cranberries) (optional)
2 teaspoons vanilla extract	
1/8 teaspoon salt	

Cut the butter into the brown sugar in a mixing bowl until crumbly. Add the skim milk, eggs, vanilla and salt gradually, beating constantly until blended. Stir in the rice. Add the lemon juice, lemon zest and dried fruit and mix well.

Spoon the rice mixture into a baking dish and bake at 325 degrees for 50 minutes. Spoon the pudding into dessert bowls. Garnish with whipped cream, ice cream and/or mashed sweetened berries.

Microwave a lemon for fifteen seconds before squeezing to double the juice.

NUTRIENTS PER SERVING • Yield: 6 servings

CAL	PROT	CARBO	T FAT	SAT. FAT	MONOUFA	FIBER	SOD	OMEGA-3 FATS	MG	K
223	8G	36G	5G	1G	2G	1G	142MG	<1G	43MG	223MG

Raisin Pudding Cake

2/3 **cup granulated sugar**	1/2 **cup skim milk**
1/2 **cup all-purpose flour**	2 **cups water**
1/2 **cup whole wheat flour**	1 **cup packed brown sugar**
11/2 **teaspoons baking powder**	2 **tablespoons butter or trans-fat-free margarine**
1/4 **teaspoon salt**	
1 **cup raisins**	

Mix the granulated sugar, all-purpose flour, whole wheat flour, baking powder and salt in a bowl. Add the raisins and stir until coated. Add the skim milk and stir just until moistened; do not overmix. Spread the batter in a 9x9-inch baking pan sprayed with nonstick cooking spray.

Combine the water, brown sugar and butter in a small saucepan and simmer just until the butter melts and the sugar dissolves, stirring frequently. Pour the butter mixture over the prepared layer; do not stir. Bake at 350 degrees for 30 to 40 minutes or until the edges pull from the sides of the pan. Serve warm, garnished with lite whipped topping and cinnamon if desired.

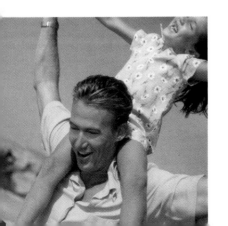

NUTRIENTS PER SERVING   Yield: 9 servings

CAL	PROT	CARBO	T FAT	SAT. FAT	MONOUFA	FIBER	SOD	OMEGA-3 FA	MG	K
273	3G	62G	3G	2G	1G	2G	181MG	<1G	25MG	262MG

Chocolate Mocha Cake

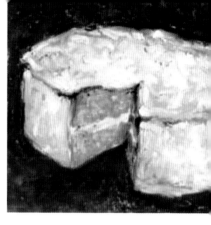

1 **cup whole wheat flour**	1 **cup sugar**
1 **cup all-purpose flour**	2 **tablespoons butter or**
2 **teaspoons baking soda**	**trans-fat-free margarine**
1 **cup (6 ounces) semisweet**	3 **Omega-3-enhanced eggs**
chocolate chips	2 **cups brewed coffee, chilled**
3 **tablespoons 1% milk**	

Mix the whole wheat flour, all-purpose flour and baking soda in a bowl. Heat the chocolate chips and 1% milk in a saucepan until blended, stirring frequently. Beat the sugar and butter in a mixing bowl until creamy, scraping the bowl occasionally. Add the eggs to the creamed mixture 1 at a time, beating well after each addition. Blend in the chocolate mixture. Add the flour mixture and coffee and beat until blended.

Spoon the batter into a 9x13-inch cake pan sprayed with nonstick cooking pray. Bake at 350 degrees for 22 to 25 minutes or until a wooden pick inserted in the center comes out clean. Cool in the pan on a wire rack. Cut into squares and garnish with fresh fruit and a dollop of lite whipped cream if desired.

To ease cutting, dip a knife in water before cutting cakes.

NUTRIENTS PER SERVING   Yield: 24 servings

CAL	PROT	CARBO	T FAT	SAT. FAT	MONOUFA	FIBER	SOD	OMEGA-3 FATS	MG	K
120	2G	21G	4G	2G	1G	1G	123MG	<1G	18MG	73MG

Buttermilk not available? Add two teaspoons of vinegar or lemon juice to each 1/2 cup of skim milk.

desserts

Chocolate Zucchini Cake

1 **cup all-purpose flour**	3/4 **cup artificial sweetener**
1 **cup whole wheat flour**	1/2 **cup unsweetened applesauce**
1/2 **cup ground flaxseed**	1/2 **cup buttermilk**
1/4 **cup unsweetened baking cocoa**	1/4 **cup canola oil**
1 **teaspoon baking soda**	2 **Omega-3-enhanced eggs**
3/4 **teaspoon ground cinnamon**	1 **teaspoon vanilla extract**
1/2 **teaspoon ground cloves**	2 **cups grated seeded unpeeled zucchini**
1/2 **teaspoon baking powder**	
1/2 **teaspoon salt**	1 **cup (6 ounces) semisweet chocolate chips**
1 **cup sugar**	

Mix the all-purpose flour, whole wheat flour, flaxseed, baking cocoa, baking soda, cinnamon, cloves, baking powder and salt in a bowl. Combine the sugar, artificial sweetener, applesauce, buttermilk, canola oil, eggs and vanilla in a mixing bowl and beat until blended, scraping the bowl occasionally. Add the zucchini and beat until incorporated. Blend in the flour mixture and stir in the chocolate chips.

Spoon the batter into a 9x13-inch cake pan sprayed with nonstick cooking spray. Bake at 350 degrees for 30 minutes or until a wooden pick inserted in the center comes out clean; the chocolate chips will stick to the wooden pick. Cool in the pan on a wire rack and cut into squares. You may freeze for future use. For variety, omit the chocolate chips from the batter and sprinkle over the top of the warm cake to self frost.

NUTRIENTS PER SERVING   Yield: 18 servings

CAL	PROT	CARBO	T FAT	SAT. FAT	MONOUFA	FIBER	SOD	OMEGA-3 FA	MG	K
227	4G	37G	8G	2G	3G	3G	168MG	1G	40MG	193MG

Cranberry Carrot Cake

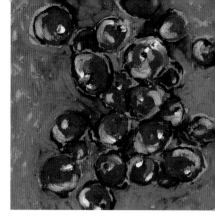

¹/2 cup drained crushed pineapple in lite syrup

³/4 cup all-purpose flour

¹/2 cup whole wheat flour

¹/4 cup ground flaxseed

2 teaspoons ground cinnamon

1 teaspoon baking soda

¹/4 teaspoon salt

¹/2 cup packed brown sugar

¹/2 cup granulated sugar or artificial sweetener

¹/4 cup canola oil

¹/4 cup unsweetened applesauce

2 Omega-3-enhanced eggs

1 teaspoon vanilla extract

3 cups grated carrots

¹/2 cup walnuts, chopped

¹/2 cup dried cranberries

¹/2 cup shredded coconut

Squeeze the excess syrup from the pineapple. Combine the all-purpose flour, whole wheat flour, flaxseed, cinnamon, baking soda and salt in a bowl and mix well. Combine the brown sugar, granulated sugar, canola oil and applesauce in a mixing bowl and beat at medium speed until blended, scraping the bowl occasionally. Add the eggs and vanilla and beat at medium speed until incorporated. Beat in the flour mixture. Add the pineapple, carrots, walnuts, cranberries and coconut and beat at low speed until combined.

Spread the batter in a full sheet pan sprayed with nonstick cooking spray. Bake at 350 degrees for 40 to 45 minutes or until a wooden pick inserted in the center comes out clean; do not overbake. Cool in the pan on a wire rack. Spread with cream cheese frosting if desired.

NUTRIENTS PER SERVING　　　　　　　　　　Yield: 18 servings

CAL	PROT	CARBO	T FAT	SAT. FAT	MONOUFA	FIBER	SOD	OMEGA-3 FATS	MG	K
168	3G	25G	7G	1G	2G	2G	127MG	1G	24MG	152MG

One-half teaspoon of cinnamon may help lower blood glucose levels by eighteen to twenty-nine percent in those who have Type 2 diabetes, and it may also help lower LDL cholesterol and triglycerides.

Cinnamon Coffee Bars

3/4 cup all-purpose flour	1 cup packed brown sugar
3/4 cup whole wheat flour	1 Omega-3-enhanced egg
1 teaspoon baking powder	1/2 cup brewed hot coffee
1/2 teaspoon ground cinnamon	1/4 cup unsweetened applesauce
1/4 teaspoon baking soda	1/2 cup raisins
1/4 teaspoon salt	1/2 cup pecans, chopped
1/4 cup (1/2 stick) butter or trans-fat-free margarine, softened	1/2 cup confectioners' sugar
	1 tablespoon milk

Mix the all-purpose flour, whole wheat flour, baking powder, cinnamon, baking soda and salt in a bowl. Combine the butter, brown sugar and egg in a mixing bowl and beat until creamy, scraping the bowl occasionally. Add the coffee and applesauce and beat until blended. Beat in the flour mixture until incorporated. Stir in the raisins and pecans.

Spoon the coffee mixture into a 9x13-inch baking dish and bake at 350 degrees for 18 to 20 minutes or until the edges pull from the sides of the pan.

Combine the confectioners' sugar and milk in a bowl and stir until of a drizzling consistency. Drizzle the icing over the warm layer. Cool in the pan on a wire rack and cut into bars. Store in an airtight container.

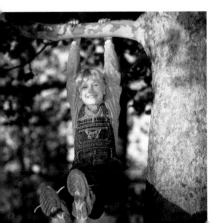

NUTRIENTS PER BAR   Yield: 1 dozen bars

CAL	PROT	CARBO	T FAT	SAT. FAT	MONOUFA	FIBER	SOD	OMEGA-3 FA	MG	K
234	3G	40G	8G	3G	3G	2G	157MG	<1G	26MG	183MG

Better-for-You Brownies

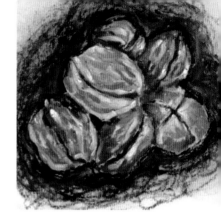

1/2 cup unsweetened baking cocoa	1/4 teaspoon salt
1/2 cup chopped pitted dates	1 cup sugar
1 teaspoon instant coffee granules	1 Omega-3-enhanced egg
1/2 cup boiling water	1 Omega-3-enhanced egg white
1/3 cup walnut halves	2 tablespoons canola oil
2/3 cup all-purpose flour	1 teaspoon vanilla extract
1/2 teaspoon baking powder	1 tablespoon sugar

Combine the baking cocoa, dates and coffee granules in a heatproof bowl. Add the boiling water and stir until the baking cocoa dissolves. Let stand for 10 minutes or until cool. Spread the walnuts in a shallow baking pan and toast at 350 degrees for 4 to 6 minutes or until light brown and fragrant, stirring occasionally. Remove the walnuts to a plate to cool. Maintain the oven temperature.

Combine the toasted walnuts, flour, baking powder and salt in a food processor and process until the walnuts are ground. Pour the walnut mixture into a large bowl. Scrape the cocoa mixture into the food processor and add 1 cup sugar, the egg, egg white, canola oil and vanilla. Process until smooth, scraping the side of the bowl once or twice. Add the cocoa mixture to the walnut mixture and stir just until moistened.

Spoon the batter into a 9x9-inch baking pan sprayed with nonstick cooking spray and sprinkle with 1 tablespoon sugar. Bake at 350 degrees for 25 to 30 minutes or until the edges are firm and just set in the center. Cool in the pan on a wire rack. Coat a sharp knife with nonstick cooking spray and cut into 16 squares. Store in an airtight container.

NUTRIENTS PER BROWNIE   Yield: 16 brownies

CAL	PROT	CARBO	T FAT	SAT. FAT	MONOUFA	FIBER	SOD	OMEGA-3 FATS	MG	K
126	2G	23G	4G	<1G	1G	2G	60MG	<1G	19MG	98MG

desserts

Gingerbread Boys

2	**cups all-purpose flour**
1/2	**cup whole wheat flour**
1/2	**teaspoon baking soda**
3/4	**teaspoon salt**
3/4	**teaspoon ground ginger**
1/4	**teaspoon ground nutmeg (optional)**

1/8	**teaspoon ground allspice**
1/2	**cup (1 stick) butter or trans-fat-free margarine, softened**
1/2	**cup sugar**
1/2	**cup dark molasses**
1/4	**cup water**

Mix the all-purpose flour, whole wheat flour, baking soda, salt, ginger, nutmeg and allspice in a bowl. Beat the butter and sugar in a mixing bowl until creamy. Add the flour mixture, molasses and water and beat until blended. Chill, covered, for 3 hours or longer.

Roll the dough 1/4 inch thick on a lightly floured surface. Cut into desired shapes and arrange 2 inches apart on a cookie sheet. Bake at 375 degrees for 8 to 10 minutes or until crisp around the edges. Cool on the cookie sheet for 2 minutes. Remove to a wire rack to cool completely.

Pipe eyes, buttons and pockets with confectioners' sugar frosting. Or you can use red hot candies and/or raisins to represent eyes and buttons. Flavor the frosting with peppermint extract if desired. Store in an airtight container.

NUTRIENTS PER COOKIE — Makes 2 dozen cookies

CAL	PROT	CARBO	T FAT	SAT. FAT	MONOUFA	FIBER	SOD	OMEGA-3 FA	MG	K
113	1G	19G	4G	2G	1G	1G	129MG	<1G	6MG	149MG

Nutritional profile does not include frosting.

Chocolate
Peanut Butter Pockets

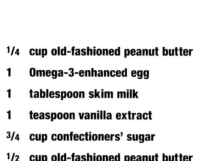

1 **cup all-purpose flour**	1/4 **cup old-fashioned peanut butter**
1/2 **cup whole wheat flour**	1 **Omega-3-enhanced egg**
1/2 **cup unsweetened baking cocoa**	1 **tablespoon skim milk**
1/2 **teaspoon baking soda**	1 **teaspoon vanilla extract**
1/2 **cup (1 stick) butter or trans-fat-free margarine, softened**	3/4 **cup confectioners' sugar**
1/2 **cup granulated sugar**	1/2 **cup old-fashioned peanut butter**
1/2 **cup packed brown sugar**	2 **tablespoons granulated sugar**

Mix the all-purpose flour, whole wheat flour, baking cocoa and baking soda in a bowl and mix well. Beat the next 4 ingredients in a mixing bowl until creamy. Add the egg, skim milk and vanilla and beat until smooth. Beat in as much of the flour mixture as possible with the mixer and beat in the remaining flour mixture by hand. Shape the chocolate dough into thirty-two 1 1/4-inch balls.

Mix the confectioners' sugar and 1/2 cup peanut butter in a mixing bowl until smooth. Shape the dough into thirty-two 3/4-inch balls. Slightly flatten 1 chocolate dough ball and top with a peanut butter ball. Shape the chocolate dough over the peanut butter dough to cover and roll into a ball. Repeat the process with the remaining chocolate dough balls and remaining peanut butter dough balls.

Arrange the dough balls 2 inches apart on an ungreased cookie sheet. Flatten lightly with the bottom of a glass dipped in 2 tablespoons granulated sugar. Bake at 350 degrees for 8 minutes or until set and slightly cracked. Cool on the cookie sheet for 1 minute. Remove to a wire rack to cool completely. Store in an airtight container.

NUTRIENTS PER COOKIE   Makes 32 cookies

CAL	PROT	CARBO	T FAT	SAT. FAT	MONOUFA	FIBER	SOD	OMEGA-3 FATS	MG	K
126	3G	16G	6G	2G	2G	1G	67MG	<1G	11MG	48MG

Cranberry Pumpkin Loaves

If you take flax oil in pills or liquid form, you miss important nutrients such as potassium, fiber, magnesium, and vitamin E found in whole flaxseed. The cholesterol-lowering benefits of flax are mostly from the fiber, not the oil.

1¹/₂ cups all-purpose flour	1¹/₂ cups artificial sweetener
1¹/₄ cups whole wheat flour	1 (15-ounce) can pumpkin
¹/₄ cup ground flaxseed	4 Omega-3-enhanced eggs
1 tablespoon plus 2 teaspoons pumpkin pie spice	¹/₂ cup canola oil
2 teaspoons baking soda	¹/₂ cup unsweetened applesauce
1¹/₂ teaspoons salt	¹/₂ cup water
1¹/₂ cups sugar	1 cup dried, fresh or frozen cranberries

Combine the all-purpose flour, whole wheat flour, flaxseed, pumpkin pie spice, baking soda and salt in a bowl and mix well. Combine the sugar, artificial sweetener, pumpkin, eggs, canola oil, applesauce and water in a mixing bowl and beat just until blended. Add the pumpkin mixture to the flour mixture and stir just until moistened. Fold in the cranberries.

Spoon equal portions of the batter into 2 greased and floured 5x9-inch loaf pans. Bake at 350 degrees for 60 to 65 minutes or until a wooden pick inserted in the centers comes out clean. Cool in the pans on a wire rack for 10 minutes. Remove to a wire rack to cool completely.

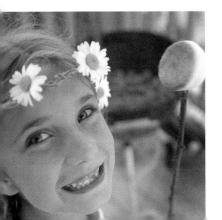

NUTRIENTS PER SLICE   Yield: 20 slices

CAL	PROT	CARBO	T FAT	SAT. FAT	MONOUFA	FIBER	SOD	OMEGA-3 FA	MG	K
226	4G	38G	7G	1G	4G	3G	317MG	1G	20MG	73MG

Key Lime Pie

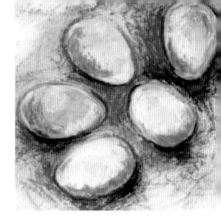

1	Walnut Crust (page 136)	4	Omega-3-enhanced egg yolks
1	(14-ounce) can fat-free sweetened condensed milk	1/2	cup lime juice
		3	to 4 teaspoons grated lime zest

Prepare and bake the Walnut Crust. Whisk the condensed milk, egg yolks, lime juice and lime zest in a bowl for 3 minutes or until thickened.

Pour the lime filling into the crust and bake at 325 degrees for 15 to 20 minutes or until the center is set. Chill, covered, for 2 hours or for up to 4 days.

NUTRIENTS PER SERVING   Yield: 10 servings

CAL	PROT	CARBO	T FAT	SAT. FAT	MONOUFA	FIBER	SOD	OMEGA-3 FATS	MG	K
249	7G	35G	9G	3G	2G	1G	75MG	1G	28MG	219MG

Walnut Crust

3/4 **cup all-purpose flour**

1/4 **cup whole wheat flour**

1/2 **cup finely chopped walnuts or nut of choice**

3 **tablespoons unsalted butter or trans-fat-free margarine, chilled and cut into small pieces**

1/8 **teaspoon salt**

2 **to 4 tablespoons cold water**

Combine the all-purpose flour, whole wheat flour, walnuts, butter and salt in a bowl and blend with a pastry cutter. Add just enough of the cold water until the dough adheres, stirring constantly with a fork.

Roll the dough on a lightly floured surface and fit into a 9-inch pie plate. Trim the edge and pierce the bottom and side with a fork. Bake at 350 degrees for 15 minutes or until light brown.

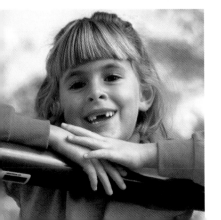

NUTRIENTS PER SERVING   Yield: 10 servings

CAL	PROT	CARBO	T FAT	SAT. FAT	MONOUFA	FIBER	SOD	OMEGA-3 FA	MG	K
114	2G	10G	7G	3G	1G	1G	30MG	1G	16MG	50MG

Olive Oil Conversions

For moist and even-textured baked goods, substitute a mild-flavored extra-light olive oil in place of butter or margarine. Olive oil adds a light delicious taste to cakes, breads, and muffins.

Butter/Margarine	Olive Oil
1 teaspoon	3/4 teaspoon
1 tablespoon	2 1/4 teaspoons
2 tablespoons	1 1/2 tablespoons
1/4 cup	3 tablespoons
1/3 cup	1/4 cup
1/2 cup	1/4 cup plus 2 tablespoons
2/3 cup	1/2 cup
3/4 cup	1/2 cup plus 1 tablespoon
1 cup	3/4 cup

Source: www.bertolli.com

Index

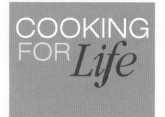

YOUR ORDER	QTY	TOTAL
Cooking for Life, Volume 2 at $19.95 per cookbook		$
Shipping and handling $5.00 for 1 book and $1.00 for each additional book shipped to the same address		$
	Subtotal	$
South Dakota residents add 6% sales tax to subtotal (no tax if mailing outside of South Dakota)	Tax	$
	Total	$

Bill to:

Name

Street Address

City   State   Zip

Telephone ( )   E-mail

Ship to: [ ] Same as billing address. (Please print. If multiple ship to addresses, please attach to this form.)

Name

Street Address

City   State   Zip

Telephone ( )   E-mail

Method of Payment: [ ] Check made payable to Avera McKennan Foundation
[ ] VISA [ ] MasterCard [ ] Discover
[ ] American Express

Name
(Print name as it appears on your charge card.)

Account #   Expiration Date (Mo/Yr)

Cardholder's Signature

Avera McKennan
Foundation
800 East 21st Street
PO Box 5045
Sioux Falls, SD
57117-5045

Place your order today!

Call: 605-322-8900

Mail this form to: Avera McKennan Foundation

Go online at www.avera mckennanfoundation.org to order COOKING FOR LIFE cookbooks and other customized gift items that are perfect for your own kitchen or the kitchen of a friend or loved one!

Cookbook sale proceeds benefit the patients of the
Avera Heart Hospital of South Dakota.

Photocopies will be accepted.

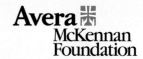

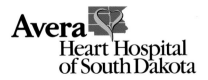

Avera
Heart Hospital
of South Dakota